PSYCHIATR
PHARMACOGENETICS
from concepts to cases

David B. Durham, MD, MPH
Ranjit K. Thirumaran, MPharm, PhD

A publication by

Fortis Caliga Academic Press

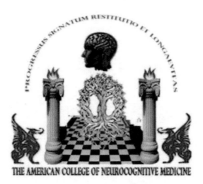

THE AMERICAN COLLEGE OF NEUROCOGNITIVE MEDICINE

TABLE OF CONTENTS

Acknowledgments 1

Prologue..3

Introduction 5

Adverse Drug Reactions - Adverse Drug Events and the Bottom Line................8

Basic Cellular Physiology of Pharmacogenetics 11

The Cytochrome P450 System 17

The Clinical Utility of Pharmacogenetics in the Context of Liability..............21

Social and Regulatory Impact of Pharmacogenetics..26

Ethical Considerations of Pharmacogenetics in Clinical Practice 28

The Current Evidence Supporting Pharmacogenetic Testing...........................30

Substrates, Inhibitors, Inducers and the Drug-Protein Complex 37

Epidemiology and Clinical Utility of the CYP2D6 Enzyme..............................41

Epidemiology and Clinical Utility of the CYP2C19 Enzyme............................49

Epidemiology and Clinical Utility of the CYP2C9 Enzyme..............................53

Epidemiology and Clinical Utility of the CYP1A2 Enzyme 57

Epidemiology and Clinical Utility of the CYP3A4 / 3A5 Enzymes...................60

Clinical Cases in Psychiatric Pharmacogenetics Cases
from the Clinic and Hospital...67

Conclusion..108

Selected Psychotropic Drugs and their Clinically Relevant
Pharmacogenetics 199 112

Major Web Sources for Pharmacogenomics 115

Bibliography..116

Historical Landmarks Leading to the Discovery of Pharmacogenetics 126

Addendum: Population, Disease-Specific, and Sequence Databases 129

End Notes..131

About the Authors 142

Acknowledgments

The authors would like to express their thanks and gratitude to the following people, without whom this book would not have been made possible: Dr. Erin Schuetz, Dr. Cezary Skobowiat, and Dr. Sanjay Bansal for their scientific inspiration; Dr. Len Del Carmen, for her editorial talent and enduring support; Dr. Herbie and Lew Goodman, for their 'New York' moxy and wisdom; the late Dr. David Mrazek, extraorindary man and psychiatrist, and pharmacogenetics pioneer; Dr. Ira Salom for his time and editorial effort; Dr. Steve Black for his humor, inspiration and friendship; Dr. Alya Reeve for her willingness to always share her wisdom with grace; Howard Coleman, Dr. Tia Aulinskas, Kristine Ashcraft, and the outstanding scientists at Genelex; the University of New Mexico Psychiatry Department; Wil Elliot and Mike Fitch, for their support, friendship and patience; Laura Jobb, for her friendship and unyielding optimism; Dr. Rob Sher, for his loyal friendship, wit and sharp mind; the late Dr. Phillip Briggs, for his creativity and inspiration; Robert Durham, for his love and friendship under any circumstances; Greg 'Nakios' Anderson, for his friendship, creativity and support when it counted the most; Molly Schmidt-Nowara, for her friendship and help in difficult times; Dr. Wil Spradlin, for his wisdom on the making and keeping of thoroughbreds; Dr. Dan Bowen and Benedictine College, where my love for genetics started; the American College of Neurocognitive Medicine for their financial support and guidance; to Ravi Ramgati, for his technical and editorial expertise and work ethic; to Dr. Steve Cain, for his fastidious eye and editorial review; to the late Bob Colby, a great writer, editor and man – you are incredibly missed; to our students, who help remind us to stay inspired; to our patients, who remind us of our duty to continually strive for safer and more precise treatment approaches; and finally, to our parents, for their encouragement and continued support.

PROLOGUE

At the completion of the Human Genome Project, the world sat in attentive expectation of new approaches to disease prevention, diagnosis and treatment that would either orbit the miraculous, or deliver it outright. This expectation is now being properly tempered by an appreciation of the extraordinary complexity of what we have learned, and the somewhat disappointing realization that we have only since developed rather blunt instruments as a result of the knowledge we gained. But some of these tools are quickly evolving and now show legitimate clinical utility. The technology of pharmacogenetic testing is one of these tools, and its relevance to the field of psychiatry is quickly taking hold.

The sub-specialty of psychiatry remains the most subjective field in medicine. This 'subjectiveness' has been one of the largest barriers to improve accuracy of diagnosis, to measurably reduce adverse drug events and substantially improve treatment outcomes. The utilization of pharmacogenetic technology in psychiatry is the first clinical modality of its kind to quantifiably increase both accuracy and precision of prescribing psychotropic medications while simultaneously reducing adverse drug events. The timing of this technology is auspicious. Psychotropic medications are now the most prescribed drugs in medicine, despite a repository of data that clearly reveals they are far from benign. Just as compelling is the data showing that nearly half of people prescribed these medications do not respond well to treatment with them. Many of these non-responding patients often require complex psychotropic cocktails which dramatically compound the potential for adverse drug events. It is, in essence, a perfect storm for pharmacogenetic technology to add substantial benefit to the field of psychiatry. There are excellent works available on the science of pharmacogenetics and its evolving technology. This book will draw from a number of these and provide the reader with a basic overview of this technology. Its purpose, however, is what its name promises: to guide the psychiatric clinician on the application of pharmacogenetic technology, and provide real-world case studies of psychiatric patients who have benefited from it.

INTRODUCTION

"Chance mutations are the raw genetic material of evolution. Environmental challenge, deciding which mutants and their combinations will survive, is the necessity that molds us further from this protean genetic clay."

Chapter 7, From Genes to Culture
Consilience: the unity of knowledge
Edwin O. Wilson, 1999

Pharmacogenetics is the study of how genetic variability alters how we respond to a drug. This relatively new field combines pharmacology (the science of drugs) and genomics (the study of genes and their functions) to help develop effective and safe medications in doses that will be tailored to an individual's unique genetic makeup. Pharmacogenetics and Pharmacogenomics are terms used interchangeably. Both terms form the basis for the concept of 'Personalized Medicine'. Technically, pharmacogenetics is associated with the study of how a drug is affected by an individual's genes, and pharmacogenomics refers to genome-wide studies of populations of genes.

The field of pharmacogenetics has its roots in the decade of the 1950s with the emergence of molecular biology after Drs. Watson and Crick published their famous article in the journal *Nature* describing, for the first time, the double helix structure of Deoxyribonucleic Acid (DNA).[1] Genetic research was catapulted to the modern age. Researchers soon discovered that certain genetic enzyme abnormalities (polymorphisms) were found to be predisposed to unexpected adverse drug reactions. An early example of this is hemolytic anemia resulting from a deficiency of the Glucose-6-phosphate dehydrogenase (G-6-PD) enzyme. A deficiency of 80 to 95 percent of this enzyme can lead to hemolytic anemia after people with this deficiency eat fava beans.[2]

The medical geneticist Lawrence Snyder is frequently recognized as the one who laid the early groundwork for the field of pharmacogenetics.

Although his studies ranged from subjects such as hemophilia, baldness and Rh incompatibility, he is best remembered for his inheritance studies of phenylthiocarbamide. He discovered that the reason this chemical is bitter to some individuals and tasteless to others depended on the autosomal recessive variant of a single gene.[3] The title of "father of modern pharmacogenetics", however, is most often attributed to Arno Motulsky who, in 1957, postulated that polymorphic variability in enzymes that metabolize drugs are important in managing drug reactions.[4][5] In 1959 the German scientist Friedrich Vogel was the first to apply the term "pharmacogenetics" and defined it as the "study of the role of genetics in drug response".[6][7] In 1962, Werner Kalow published one of the first modern systemic account of drugs and their metabolism: *Pharmacogenetics – the Heredity and the Response to Drugs.*[8] In 1968, Swedish researcher Folker Sjöqvist and his team established that the metabolism of tricylic antidepressants is under genetic control.[9] That same year E.S. Vesell showed remarkable similarity in drug elimination for several drugs in identical twins – most notably with *phenylbutazone.*[10] In the 1980s, the field of pharmacogenetics gained more momentum with a number of landmark discoveries. These include the discovery of the genetic polymorphism of thiopurine-methyltransferase (TPMT) by Weinshilboum and Sladek in 1980 – which holds clinical significance for drugs such as 6-mercaptopurine and others used as chemotherapeutic agents and the description of the polymorphism of mephenytoin hydroxylation by Kupfer and Wedlund in 1984 – which is important for persons on Phenytoin for seizure control. In 1986 Dr. Kary Mullis introduced the polymerase chain reaction technique which allowed the exponential amplification of genetic sequences.[11] In 1991, the first issue of the journal *Pharmacogenetics* was published. Finally, over the past two decades, and turbo charged by the mapping of the human genome, our discoveries have resulted in pharmacogenetics now being utilized as a clinical tool.

Science appears to have arisen as the champion in bringing pharmacogenomics to the eyes and ears of market forces, who have begun to view it as a value-added biotechnology. This new 'tool' is slowly gaining ground even with insurance payers. Insurance payers are beginning to understand, albeit slowly, that pharmacogenetic technology can provide exceptional clinical value to the well-versed practitioner as it stratifies individuals into predictable categories of response to a drug, thereby improving clinical outcomes and safety while reducing long-term cost and, in addition, reducing clinician liability. Pharmacogenetic testing returns actionable information to the clinician on how a medication will be uniquely utilized by a specific individual.[12]

The most important of the 'actionable information' for clinicians is packaged as the *phenotype*. The phenotype is defined as the outward, physical manifestation of an organism. The *genotype*, by contrast, is the internally coded, inheritable information contained in DNA, which holds the critical instructions that are used and interpreted by the molecular machinery of cells. The passage of time with the resulting physiologic aberrations known as aging, and the exposure to the unique mosaic of each individual's environment, is the part of the equation needed to form an individual's phenotype. Thus, the phenotype is a prediction of how a particular person, built by genetic programming, will perform in an environment. A practical example is a seven foot male. The genotype of this male codes for a height of 7 feet. His phenotype is analogous to, for example, how he is predicted to perform on the basketball court. The use of new biostatistical, biotechnological and computational tools to develop the phenotype from the genotype is slowly increasing in sophistication. The process of developing phenotype models in pharmacogenetics, however, does remain a challenge as its precision, accuracy and 'actionability' is directly related to how well our current science is able to make predictions. If a clinician orders pharmacogenetic testing on an individual, the quantifiable accuracy and value of the data he receives is not simply dependent on the number of known genes and the variability in their respective alleles. Accurately developing a person's phenotype must also consider ethnicity, sex, age, tobacco and other chemical use – in addition to co-medications – and a subject's history of response to treatment. The good news is that with broader and more frequent use of pharmacogenetic testing, and the broader advancements in the science of human genetics, the precision and accuracy of phenotype development is improving.[13] Finally, the creation of a unified central pharmacogenomic information repository has yet to occur. The creation of such a database would certainly enhance the precision of pharmacogenetic testing and greatly further this science as the predictability of responding to a given medication as well as suffering adverse reactions would be exponentially enhanced.

ADVERSE DRUG REACTIONS - ADVERSE DRUG EVENTS AND THE BOTTOM LINE

Adverse drug reactions (ADRs) are a significant cause of hospitalizations and deaths in the United States. An ADR is defined as "Harm caused by a drug with normal use, that is not expected"; whereas an Adverse Drug Event (ADE) is more broadly defined as "Harm caused by use of a drug or inappropriate use of a drug". ADEs and other drug-related problems are a risk of major concern, particularly amongst elderly and polypharmacy-treated patients where the incidence of major iatrogenic events is estimated to reach more than 25 percent. [14] [15] [16] [17] [18] In 2009 alone, the Centers for Disease Control have estimated that more than 700,000 emergency room visits were for ADRs in Medicare patients alone. It is currently estimated that approximately 8 percent of all healthcare costs are related to the adverse impact of prescription drugs. The cost of managing ADRs is extraordinary. In 2012, the Centers for Medicaid and Medicare Services estimated it spent $3.8 billion in managing ADRs. Research has shown that 16.6 percent of hospitalizations in the elderly are due to ADRs.[19] Many ADEs result from variations in the CYP450 enzymes, making the ability to detect variations in these genes all the more important. Current meta-data estimates that approximately 46 percent of ADRs are preventable.

With the knowledge gained from the Human Genome Project, science has gained significant momentum in learning how inherited differences in genes affect the body's response to medications. These genetic differences can now be used to predict whether a medication will be effective for an individual and help reduce and prevent ADRs. Because an estimated 70 percent of psychotropic medications are metabolized by a handful of Cytochromes – the metabolizing enzymes for most drugs in the liver and intestine – the scope of research has been sufficiently narrowed to determine what enzymes metabolize what drug. The most common Cytochromes that metabolize medications are CYP2D6, CYP2C19,

CYP2C9, CYP3A4, CYP3A5 and CYP1A2. These, and other enzymes in this family, can now be measured utilizing common laboratory techniques. Thus, the bedside utility of pharmacogenetic technology in psychiatry has come of age. Its clinical value is accelerating as it holds promise to be one of the most effective and efficient empirical tools to predict and manage ADRs arising from psychotropic medications to date.

> *In 2012, the Centers for Medicaid and Medicare Services estimated it spent $3.8 billion in managing ADRs.*

The adoption of a new technology in medicine today is dependent on its ability to positively affect the bottom line. Data from the National Institute of Health's Clinical Pharmacogenetics Implementation Consortium as well as private institutions have shown that, when pharmacogenetic testing is correctly applied, the savings can be dramatic over the moderate and long term. The emergence of scientific leaders who champion pharmacogenetic technology is providing some of the needed momentum for its wider adoption. Dr. Richard Weinshilboum has been one of these champions for many years. He is a highly distinguished medical scientist at the Mayo Clinic who has studied inheritance and individual variation in DNA and drug response. In his March 2011 article in the New England Journal of Medicine titled Genomic Medicine, he writes:

> *"The promise of pharmacogenetics, the study of the role of inheritance in the individual variation in drug response, lies in its potential to identify the right drug and dose for each patient. Even though individual differences in drug response can result from the effects of age, sex, disease or drug interactions, genetic factors also influence the efficacy of a drug and the likelihood of an adverse reaction."*

Psychiatric Pharmacogenetics is the study of how gene variants influence the responses of patients to treatment with psychotropic medications. The goal of psychiatric pharmacogenetic testing is to use genetic information to minimize the potential adverse effects of psychotropic medications and the capability to detect actual psychiatric medications that will have a high possibility of being effective for an individual patient.

The occurrence of an ADR or ADE is the end of a complex mosaic of many biochemical steps. Co-administered medications, environmental agents, diet, vitamin supplements, tobacco, and alcohol are all known to induce or inhibit Cytochrome P450 enzymes. In addition, other drug-metabolizing enzymes (such as P-Glycoprotein) as well as protein drug transporters (such as the glucose transporter GLUT1 and the renal proximal tubular urate efflux transporter ABCG2) are known to alter drug efficacy, and to induce drug-drug and drug-protein interactions. An individual's physiology including co-morbid diseases, age, sex, body weight, immune function, pregnancy, exercise, starvation, and circadian rhythm, can also contribute significantly to the individual variability of effect of prescribed drugs. That being said, Cytochrome P450 enzymes still remain a very attractive and useful biomarker because, albeit highly polymorphic in nature, they are fairly easy to identify and measure, and, with the continuous advancements in the science of genetics, increasingly more predictable in their behaviors.

The current methods to detect Adverse Drug Events (ADE) miss more than a third of potential drug interactions, masked due to unknown patient genetics. The FDA recommends that Drug-Gene Interactions (DGI) should be considered as important *as* Drug-Drug Interactions (DDI). It is shown that a combined 34 percent of all potential clinically significant drug interactions were due to Drug-Gene and Drug-Drug-Gene Interactions (DDGI).[20] Variance in drug levels presents a major therapeutic problem in dosage optimization.[21] Having readily available information about patient's genetic variations in metabolism can help significantly reduce the incidence of adverse drug reactions and allow proper dosage adjustments thereby improving response to treatment.

BASIC CELLULAR
PHYSIOLOGY OF PHARMACOGENETICS

Despite the variability of how each of us responds to medications, to alcohol, to food, to sunlight, to darkness, to variations in our skin color and our ethnicity, we are greater-than 99 percent the same in our DNA. The differences between the roughly one percent remaining are described as genetic variation. This variation mostly arises over longer periods of time, occurring principally as a phenomenon called genetic drift. Genetic drift is defined essentially as genes moving through populations. It is the basic mechanism behind evolution. This is what has occurred with the Influenza virus. Some strains have become less virulent to us because of both small changes to our human DNA over time and changes to the Influenza virus DNA over time. Some changes have become more virulent because of the very same duality occurring. Sometimes there is a phenomenon called genetic shift, which is a phenomenon that occurs over much shorter periods of time. An example of which is an Influenza strain becoming suddenly more virulent, such as the H1N1 Avian Influenza strain. Essentially, a strain that once made only birds sick, shared some DNA in a relatively short period of time with an Influenza strain that makes us sick, thus triggering a genetic shift, and the emergence of a disease which is much more toxic, and more deadly, to humans. It is the phenomenon of genetic shift that occurred in the great influenza pandemic of 1918 and most other world-wide epidemics throughout history.

The basic code of life is contained in DNA. A DNA molecule has a helix shape. Engineers often refer to a helix as a coil. In architecture, a helix is a curve by which the tangent of the curve makes a constant angle with a fixed line. It is one of the most stable, and beautiful, pieces of architecture, and is replicated in the spiral staircases seen around the world. In nature, it has extraordinary versatility in its physics of movement. Each DNA molecule consists of two helixes bonded to each other by four subunits. This is called a DNA double helix molecule. Each subunit of a DNA molecule is called a nucleotide. There are four nucleotides in total. Each form an important column of stability in the DNA helix, and they are also referred to as 'complementary bases', 'base pairs' or 'nucleotide base pairs'. The nucleotide A is for Adenine, G is for Guanine, C is for Cytosine, and T is for Thymine. Thus, each strand – or stair if you will – of the double helix DNA molecule are interspersed generally as spiraling bonds between A, T, C and G. When the DNA is healthy, and has no mutations, the bonds fall in their respective sequence of A with T and C with G.

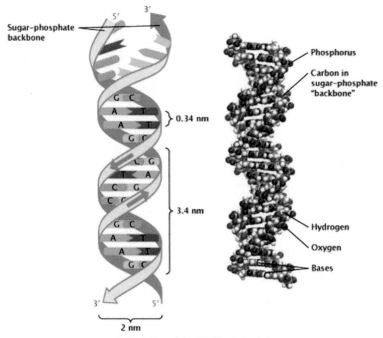

DNA Double Helix Model

Genetic variations are amongst the most essential biological differences that define inter-individual variability. The variations we are most concerned with in pharmacogenetics is a change in the DNA by just one of the nucleotide base pairs, such as C replacing T at some point. This is aptly called a single nucleotide polmorphism, or SNP, pronounced 'SNIP'. A SNP can result in a different protein and can adversely alter an enzyme's function. The definition of a SNP is a single nucleotide substitution that occurs in a population at a frequency of at least 1%. If a single nucleotide substitution occurs in less-than 1% of the population, it is referred to as a *mutation*. If the SNP results in an amino acid change, it is described as a *nonsynonymous* SNP. If, despite the nucleotide substitution, the codon codes for the same amino acid, it is described as a synonymous SNP. The SNP located in the intronic region that does not involve itself in coding is referred as an intronic SNP. The National Center for Biotechnology Information assigns a unique reference sequence number (i.e., rs number) of each variant documented. The rs number is also called the "rsSNP ID". There is also a growing understanding of genomic changes that can alter the chemistry and structure of DNA without altering its sequence though modifications such as adding single-carbon methyl groups to the DNA chain. These "epigenetic" changes can occur in response to environments and lifestyles, and influence whether certain genes are turned "on" or "off." They represent an area of intense study and have already been linked to heart disease, diabetes, and cancer. The NIH Roadmap Epigenomics Program and the Epigenetics Consortium were set up to identify this supplemental "parts list" of the human genome. [22]

Cytochromes are a family of proteins whose function is enzymatic. An enzyme is a protein that catalyzes – changes – something and has three characteristics. First, the basic function of an enzyme is to speed up a cellular reaction. In fact, enzymes speed up cellular reactions about a million times faster than they would if the enzyme were absent. Second, most enzymes are pretty specific and act with only one cellular reactant, called a substrate, to produce a product. The third, and most remarkable, characteristic of enzymes is that they are regulated in such a genetically elegant way that they are able to receive genetic program changes to go from a state of low activity to a state of high activity, and a state of high activity to low activity quite rapidly. Enzymes can catalyze a reaction at a speed of about one-hundred thousand cellular products per minute, then receive a signal that instantly increases their catalyzing speed to one-million products per minute, and then slow back down in just the same way.

A person's DNA is made up of two sets of DNA – one from each parent. This produces two sets of Cytochrome (CYP) proteins. One parent may pass along DNA that will code for a Cytochrome P450 2D6 enzyme that has normal function, and the other parent may pass along DNA that will code for a Cytochrome P450 2D6 enzyme that has a SNP that makes it half as effective of the first parent's normal P450 2D6 enzyme. Their child would then inherit a CYP2D6 enzyme with reduced function. This scenario applies, of course, to all of the CYP 450 enzymes – to include CYP2C19, CYP2C9, CYP3A4, CYP1A2, to name just a few.

It is very important, however, to note that a person's genotype may or may not result in an abnormal change in a specific CYP P450 enzyme. As mentioned before, a person's clinical phenotype is a prediction of how a person's enzyme will function given his or her genotype *and* factors such as their environment, smoking, other drugs, weight, age, ethnicity, etc. Thus, labeling a person a Poor Metabolizer, Normal Metabolizer, an Intermediate Metabolizer, or an Ultra-Rapid Metabolizer is *an educated prediction* of how they will metabolize a drug most of the time with a certain enzyme.

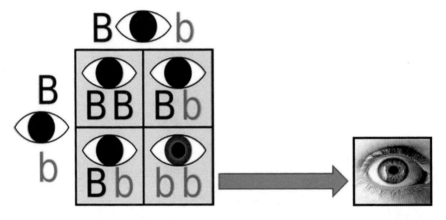

Eye color results from a rather complex interplay of genes. Two important loci are located on Chromosomes 15 and 19. Blue eyes are produced only with two blue eye genes. All four gene alleles must be blue to produce a blue eyed phenotype. Blue eye color is, thus, a recessive trait.

For example, in the case of CYP2D6, certain alleles – one of two or more alternative forms of a gene that arise by mutation and are found at the same place on a chromosome – are characterized either as wild-type alles, reduced function alleles, increased function alleles and non-functional alleles. The wild-type alleles will encode for CYP2D6 enzymes that will have normal metabolic activity; the reduced function alleles will encode for CYP2D6 enzymes that have less metabolic activity than wild-type alleles; and the non-functional alleles will encode for CYP2D6 enzymes that have little or no metabolic activity. For instance, if both parents are CYP2D6 Intermediate Metabolizers (functional/non-functional allele), their kids could either be Normal Metabolizer (functional/functional),

Intermediate Metabolizer or Poor Metabolizer (non-functional /non-functional allele).

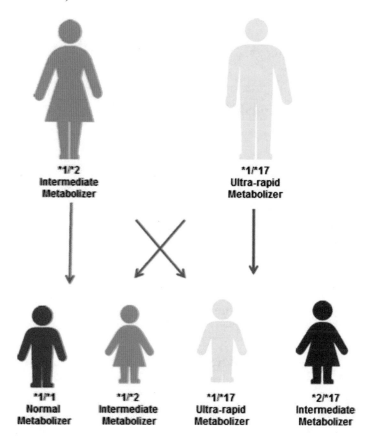

The table below summarizes the effects of cytochrome variation on therapeutic efficacy. For example, poor metabolizers are unable to metabolize certain drugs efficiently, resulting in a potentially toxic build-up of an active drug or the lack of conversion of a prodrug into an active metabolite. In contrast, in ultra-rapid metabolizers, an active drug is inactivated quickly, leading to a sub therapeutic response, while a prodrug is quickly metabolized, leading to rapid onset of therapeutic effect.

Effects of CYP variants on therapeutic efficacy

Phenotype	Active drug (inactivated by metabolism)	Prodrug (needs metabolism to produce active metabolite)
Poor Metabolizer	Increased efficacy; active metabolite may accumulate; usually require lower dose to avoid toxic accumulation	Decreased efficacy; prodrug may accumulate; may require lower dose to avoid toxic accumulation, or may require alternate drug
Ultra-Rapid Metabolizer	Decreased efficacy; active metabolite rapidly inactivated; usually require higher dose to offset inactivation	Increased efficacy; rapid onset of effect; may require lower dose to prevent excessive accumulation of active metabolite

THE CYTOCHROME P450 SYSTEM

Cytochrome noun

Biochemistry

> *any of a number of compounds consisting of heme bonded to a protein. Cytochromes function as electron transfer agents in many metabolic pathways, especially cellular respiration.*

- Oxford English Dictionary

The function of the enzymes in the Cytochrome P450 family are essential to life. On a daily basis, the human body faces a tsunami of carbon-rich, toxic compounds – From the foods we eat, to the air we breathe, to the poisons that come in contact with our skin. To prevent the poisonous accumulation of these carbon-rich toxins, the Cytochrome P450 system takes these molecules and makes them more soluble (lipophilic) which in turn allows the human body to more easily eliminate them. There are approximately fifty different Cytochrome P450 enzymes. Each of them has different functions. They are comprised of an iron atom held in a heme structure. The iron atom uses electrons to charge an oxygen atom, thus making it highly reactive. In this state, a Cytochrome P450 enzyme attacks and destroys thousands of different molecules that are toxic to our body.[23] Cytochrome P450 enzymes conduce phase I, or oxidative, metabolism as opposed to phase II conjugation.

Cytochromes (CYPs) are primarily located in our liver and the mucosal surface of the intestinal tract. They are also located in the mucosal lining of our noses. There are four CYPs that metabolize almost all drugs that pass through the liver. They are CYP2D6, CYP2C9, CYP2C19 and CYP3A4/5. Important for psychiatry, the first three of these – CYP2D6, CYP2C9 and CYP2C19 – metabolize approximately 70 percent of all psychotropic medications. Metadata from Genelex Corporation in Seattle indicates over seventy-five percent of people in North America have an abnormal variation in at least one CYP and do not metabolize medications normally.[24] It is clinically relevant and interesting to note that variations in

Cytochrome enzymes are more numerous than common genetic disorders, to include the CF carrier trait in Cystic Fibrosis, the BRCA 1 & 2 mutations in familial breast cancer, as well as Trisomy 21, or Downs Syndrome. [25]

How CYP P450 Enzymes Work

Cytochrome P450 Enzymes and their Regulation

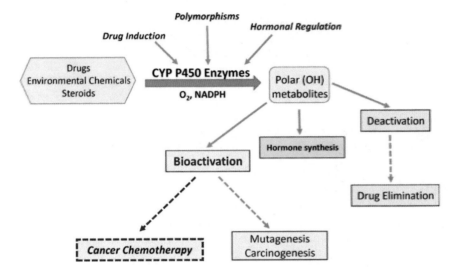

The charts below shows the average CYP P450 content in the human proximal small intestine and liver.[26] The percent contributions of individual P450 enzymes are based on total immunoquantified CYP P450 content. The values were derived from Shimada et al, (1994).[27]

Average CYP450 content in the human proximal small intestine

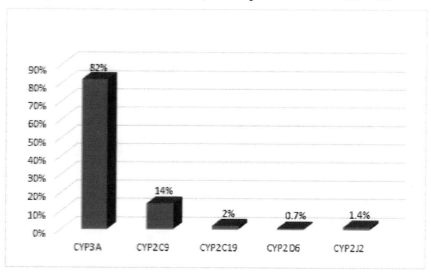

Average CYP P450 content in the human liver

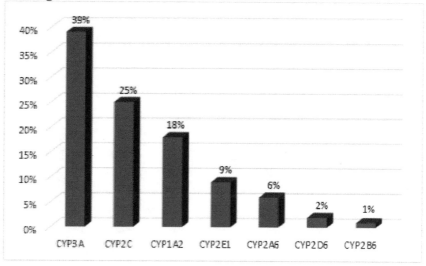

The graph below shows the number of known SNPs per CYPD6, CYP3A4, CYP1A2, CYP2C9, CYP2C19 and CYP3A5.[28]

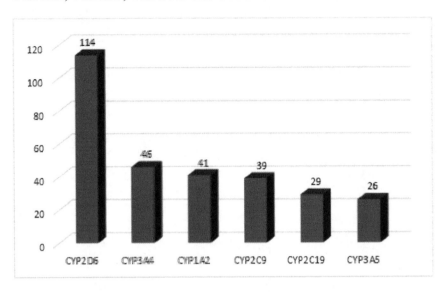

This next graph shows the number of drugs metabolized by CYPD6, CYP3A4, CYP1A2, CYP2C9, CYP2C19 and CYP3A5.[29]

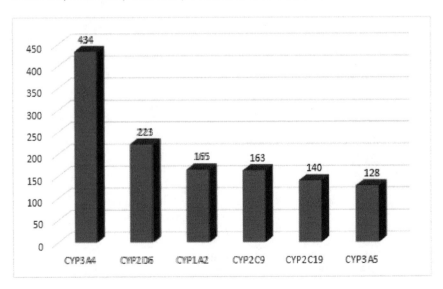

THE CLINICAL UTILITY
OF PHARMACOGENETICS
IN THE CONTEXT OF LIABILITY

P harmacogenetic testing is now a valid empirical means to increase the precision and accuracy of prescribing psychotropic medication by reducing the traditional, inefficient and often ineffective trial and error prescribing traditional to psychiatry. The appropriate use of pharmacogenetic technology can significantly reduce the incidence of adverse drug reactions as well as help reduce psychiatric practitioners' risk of legal and regulatory action. The late Dr. David Mrazek, professor of psychiatry and pediatrics and chair of the department of psychiatry and psychology at the Mayo Clinic, repeatedly acknowledged that pharmacogenetic testing in psychiatry is not only clinically useful, but more often clinically necessary. In his 2010 book *Psychiatric Pharmacoge-nomics*, Dr. Mrazek's support for pharmacogenetics is compelling:

> *"Unfortunately, the need for pharmacogenomic autopsies has
> developed as a consequence of the resistance of some physicians
> to order appropriate pharmacogenomic testing in their living
> patients."*

Psychiatrists at the Mayo Clinic have, for many years, regularly used pharmacogenetic tests to guide their prescribing of psychotropic medications.[30] The average cost of pharmacogenetic testing for each Cytochrome enzyme ranges from $100 to $300.[31]

Differences between individuals' ability to metabolize drugs are caused primarily by genetic and environmental factors. [32] An example of this can be seen in assessing the following drug toxicity scenario: a 9-year old boy, diagnosed with attention-deficit hyperactivity disorder, obsessive-compulsive disorder, and Tourette's syndrome, was treated with methylphenidate, clonidine and fluoxetine. Over a 10-month period, he developed gastrointestinal pain, poor coordination, disorientation, and seizures. He then died from a cardiac arrest. His postmortem toxicology panel showed high fluoxetine and norfluoxetine concentration. Postmortem pharmacogenetics results revealed a poor CYP2D6 metabolizer phenptype, resulting in Fluoxetine accumulation and toxicity.[33] The boy's parents were exonerated from allegations they mismanaged his medication. This technology essentially saved these unfortunate parents from going to prison. As more practitioners become aware that pharmacogenetic testing can significantly improve both accuracy and precision of prescribed psychotropic medications, as well as help reduce the traditional trial and error treatment approach now infamous in psychiatry, the number of practitioners using this new technology is increasing. Given the very robust social and regulatory pressure for improved safeguards on prescription drugs, it is likely the use of pharmacogenetic technology will only continue to increase.

> *Given that nearly one in five commonly prescribed drugs now has a pharmacogenetics warning on its package insert, practitioners increasingly have a duty to learn, understand and apply pharmacogenetic technology in their clinical practice.*

It is important for the psychiatric clinician utilizing pharmacogenetic technology to have a good understanding of the epidemiology of Cytochrome P450 variability as it is one of the most important pieces of information to justify ordering a test. The development of functional P450 activity is traditionally viewed as being limited in newborns but increasing in the first year of life to levels in toddlers and older children that generally exceed adult capacity. It is becoming apparent, however, that not all P450 enzymes share the same developmental profile and that the contribution of individual pathways to overall drug biotransformation will change with age. [34]

The enzyme developmental pattern of CYP2D6 is very low to absent in the fetus. Rapid acquisition of activity occurs as early as 2 weeks of age, so that phenotype and genotype are concordant. By age 10 years, the activity of CYP2D6 is similar to that in adults. CYP3A4 fetal activity ranges from 30-75 percent of adult values. CYP3A4 activity increases throughout infancy; by 1 year of age the activity of CYP3A4 may exceed adult values and continues at these values until early childhood or adolescence, depending on the substrate. CYP3A4 activity decreases gradually to adult levels by the end of puberty. CYP1A2 has very little activity in the fetus with acquisition of adult activity by 4-5 months of age. Activity may exceed adult rates during early childhood and decline to adult levels by the end of puberty. The CYP2C9 activity is low at birth with rapid increase in its activity that exceeds adult values during late infancy to early childhood. CYP2C9 activity then declines to adult values at the end of puberty.[35] CYP2C19 activity increases quickly after birth and reaches adult levels at approximately 6 months of age. As is the case for CYP2C9, genotype-phenotype concordance is expected at this point and predictive relationships appear between the CYP2C19 genotype and the activity of the enzyme.[36]

For the past few years, the Federal Drug Administration has strongly encouraged inclusion of pharmacogenetic data in new drug development.[37] Pharmacogenetic studies can be used at various stages of drug development. The effect of drug target polymorphisms on drug response can be assessed and identified. In clinical studies, pharmacogenetic tests can be used to stratify patients into groups based on their genotype, which corresponds to their metabolizing capacity. It can help differentiate responder populations and identify high-risk groups. This prevents the occurrence of severe adverse drug reactions and helps in better outcome of clinical trials. In addition, this can reduce attrition of drug compounds. One good example of this is the drug Abacavir, which is used in the treatment of Human Immunodeficiency Virus. Pharmacogenetic technology has been instrumental is its success. Serious and sometimes fatal hypersensitivity reactions from Abacavir were reported in approximately 8% of the patients in nine clinical trials.

Tort law in the United States has been more frequently including genetic information in pharmaceutical and medical liability cases.[38] The *state of the art* legal defense essentially considers a pharmaceutical manufacturer's decision not to warn patients in light of the technology available to them *at the time of drug approval*.[39] The technology of pharmacogenetics is now readily available, and will soon be considered, in legal terms, state of the art. It is already being utilized on a regular basis by the Food and Drug Administration and the National Institutes of Health as part of their re-consideration protocols for drugs. In their 2010 article "The Path to Personalized Medicine" in the *New England Journal of Medicine*, Dr. Margaret Hamburg, commissioner of the U.S. Food and Drug Administration, and Dr. Francis Collins, director of the National Institutes of Health, emphasize the important role now placed on genetics to bring greater precision to drug safety:

> *"As the field advances, we expect to see more efficient clinical trials based on a more thorough understanding of the genetic basis of disease. We also anticipate that some previously failed medications will be recognized as safe and effective and will be approved for subgroups of patients with specific genetic markers."* [40]

Liability is most often passed on to practicing clinicians via the law's *Learned Intermediary Doctrine.* The rationale behind this rule of law states that the medical professionals responsible for providing prescriptions are the only parties who have the necessary expertise, skill, and judgment to weigh the risks and benefits of prescribing a drug to a patient.[41] In 1999, the FDA expanded the ability of drug manufacturers to market directly to consumers. Very soon thereafter, and using the FDA's ruling, the New Jersey Supreme Court made an eye-opening ruling that limited the applicability of the Learned Intermediary Doctrine in that state.[42] With the New Jersey case as their precedent, the West Virginia Supreme Court made a similar ruling in 2007.[43] Despite these two important rulings, there have been no others. In fact, the burden of liability for adverse drug reactions still clearly remain with physicians, advanced practice nurses and physician assistants. Given that nearly one in five commonly prescribed drugs now has a pharmacogenetics warning on its package insert, practitioners increasingly have a duty to learn, understand and apply pharmacogenetic technology in their clinical practice.

It is well-known that medical liability concerns have dramatically impacted physicians. The phenomenon of "defensive medicine" is now pervasive as liability is now a multi-front threat – from lawyers to governmental regulatory bodies – such as medical boards – to advocacy groups. No longer can psychiatrists simply use their best subjective judgment in a process of trial and error for prescribing psychotropic medications. Whether this process is scientifically expedient is less a concern than whether it is *perceivably* too risky in the opinion of society, the medical boards and the social microcosm called 'the media'. It is a sad fact that psychiatrists – and physicians and even mid-level providers in general – are now guilty until proven innocent. It is, nonetheless, a fact.

It should always be remembered that the standard of care is established by a court. Plaintiff's lawyers help to establish this by calling expert witnesses to testify. Personalized justice is increasingly more frequently addressing the effect of antidepressants and/or antipsychotics on behavioral changes. Researchers have examined the relationship of violent behavior to the antidepressants paroxetine, sertraline and fluoxetine. Different verdicts in a series of medicolegal cases have reflected the different judicial processes.[44] Scientists have studied patients medicated with antidepressants and antipsychotics metabolized by polymorphic Cytochromes, and assessed the development of akathisia, suicidal and/or homicidal ideations, and their relationship to Cytochrome gene variations. The authors suggest that the key lies in understanding the interplay between the subject's CYP450 genotype, substrate drugs and doses, co-prescribed inhibitors, inducers and the age of the subject.[45] In 2009, the American Medical Association (AMA) estimated that only about 13 percent of physicians were utilizing pharmacogenetic tests in their practice.[46] In its study, the AMA did not differentiate between specialties. Today, the use of pharmacogenetic technology in psychiatric practice is increasingly more common. Moreover, there are more patients – and, thus, more jurors – aware of pharmacogenetic testing. Court cases invoking pharmacogenetic technology are increasing because the *Reasonable Person Doctrine* is, more and more, being utilized by sharp malpractice lawyers as a means to hobble a clinician being cross-examined. If a reasonable person could be expected to order a pharmacogenetic test to help reduce adverse drug reactions and improve outcomes, then a psychiatrist most definitely would be expected to do so. It is clear that the appropriate, and arguably even regular, use of pharmacogenetic technology in clinical practice is an excellent empirical method to reduce the individual and collective medical liability of not only psychiatrists, but other specialists and mid-level practitioners as well.

SOCIAL AND REGULATORY
IMPACT OF PHARMACOGENETICS

"Landmark studies...have served to open the door to the era of personalized medicine, in which doctors will use genetic information to make sure that each patient receives the right drug at the right dose at the right time."

Francis Collins, M.D., Ph.D.
Director, National Institutes of Health
2013 Mayo Clinic Leadership Conference in Pharmacogenomics

The Centers for Medicaid and Medicare Services estimate that Adverse Drug Events (ADEs) in the US cost about $289 billion per year.[47] [48] And this figure does not consider data from numerous private insurance companies.[49] Over 770,000 people are injured or die each year in hospitals from adverse drug events. Adverse drug reactions are estimated to be responsible for an estimated 100,000 deaths every year and range from the 4th to the 6th leading cause of death in the US.[50] Studies of geriatric outpatients have found the percentage of potential clinically significant adverse drug reactions ranges from 6 percent to 25 percent.[51] An estimated seventeen percent of the top 200 prescribed drugs in 2012 have an FDA pharmacogenetic warning in the package insert.

The NIH has created the Genetic Testing Registry (GTR) to provide some transparency for molecular tests offered by clinical laboratories.[52] It provides a central location for voluntary submission of genetic test information by providers. The scope includes the test's purpose, methodology, validity, evidence of the test's usefulness, and laboratory contacts and credentials. The GTR contains more than 16,000 tests from nearly 400 labs. The genetic variations in Cytochromes impact more patients than common genetic disorders. These include Trisomy 21 – aka Down's Syndrome – which occurs in 1 out of about 700 US births; Cystic Fibrosis, which occurs in about one in thirty-one people or one-thousand babies born each year; and familial breast cancer BRCA 1 and 2 which occurs in about one in eight women. Data from the Mayo Clinic, Genelex Corporation and the National Institutes of Health's Clinical

Pharmacogenetics Implementation Consortium (aka "CPIC") estimates that 75 percent of people in North America have variations in at least one of the principal CYP enzymes and do not metabolize medication normally.[53] [54]

> *Pharmacogenetics holds strong promise to improve the process of drug development as well as enhance the safe use of drugs after they are approved. It is a technology that can help revitalize a bureaucratic process that is often contrary to good medicine.*

The financial and health costs of ADRs are staggering. The FDA has, unfortunately, become overly-politicized and, thus, often appears antagonistic to an efficient and effective new drug development process. In addition, they often appear overly punitive in the post development (phase IV) process. The sad fact is that good drugs that show very good promise are often not even making it to market. A medicine that may show weaker efficacy in a more generalized patient population may show greater benefits when its use is limited to genetically defined patient populations. The lung cancer drug Iressa (gefitinib) did not demonstrate a survival advantage in a general population of patients in clinical trials, and was withdrawn from the market after initially being granted accelerated approval. The sponsoring company, however, has been using pharmacogenetics to demonstrate benefit in about 10 percent of patients who test positive for epidermal growth factor mutations, and it has won approval as a first-line treatment for that patient population in the United Kingdom. Pharmacogenetics holds strong promise to improve the process of drug development as well as enhance the safe use of drugs after they are approved.

ETHICAL CONSIDERATIONS
OF PHARMACOGENETICS
IN CLINICAL PRACTICE

Good clinicians often hold quite different values. These values are mostly shaped and defined by the environments and cultures they practice in. Fortunately, the ethical issues that psychiatric clinicians must consider when ordering pharmacogenetic tests are essentially the same as when they order other tests or labs. The two essential purposes of pharmacogenetic testing in psychiatry is to a) minimize adverse drug reactions and b) optimize the selection and dosing of psychotropic medications. When this technology is utilized correctly, it allows for a third benefit of c) reducing a clinician's liability. Although this technology operates in a very well-defined niche in medicine, it does fall under the greater umbrella of human genetics – of which history has shown its dark side.

This dark side emerged as the *eugenics* movement.[55] State legislation once provided for the sterilization of persons having presumed genetic "defects". These included mental retardation, 'incurable' mental disease, epilepsy, and even blindness and hearing loss. The first sterilization law was enacted in the State of Indiana in 1907. By 1981, a majority of States enacted sterilization laws to "correct" apparent genetic traits or their manifestations. Many of these State laws have since been repealed, and most States have amended their constitutions to mandate due process and equal protection of persons suffering from genetic disorders.

Although genes appear to yield facially neutral markers, many genetic conditions and disorders are epidemiologically tied to gender, race and ethnic groups. In particular, the prevalence of a genetic disorder among different races and ethnic groups has historically caused stigmatization and discrimination. In the United States, this form of discrimination was evident as late as the 1970s, at which time programs were enacted to screen and identify carriers of sickle cell anemia – which afflicts persons of African ethnicity. States began to enact legislation mandating genetic screening of all African Americans for sickle cell anemia, leading to discrimination and unnecessary fear. To address this, Congress in 1972 passed the National Sickle Cell Anemia Control Act, which withholds Federal funding from States unless sickle cell testing is voluntary.

As the role of genetics in medicine has become more prominent, genetic privacy has come into sharper focus. The knowledge of a person's susceptibility to disease, even before he or she shows signs or symptoms, can be a powerful tool in improving health and quality of life - but it can also be a means to discriminate in the workplace. The information could be used to limit access to insurance and other resources. To the extent that laws can confine genetic and other predictive medical information to decisions benefiting patients and their medical care, those laws will enable rather than inhibit the adoption of personalized medicine.[56] In 2008, the US Congress enacted The Genetic Nondiscrimination in Health Insurance Act (GINA). Title I of this law prohibits health plans and issuers from using genetic information to make eligibility, coverage, underwriting[57] or premium-setting decisions about covered individuals[58], even if the plan obtained the information prior to the enactment of GINA.[59] Health plans and issuers generally may not request or require that covered individuals undergo genetic testing or provide genetic information, subject to three primary exceptions.[60] The first exception is for purposes of determining the medical appropriateness of covered items and services.[61] Plans may only use the minimum amount of genetic information necessary to make such a determination. The second exception allows plans to request, in writing, that an individual voluntarily provide genetic information for research purposes, if the request explicitly states that non-compliance will not impact the individual's enrollment, premium or contribution amounts and that no information will be used for underwriting purposes.[62] The third and final exception is an "incidental collection" exception that applies when the plan obtains genetic information ancillary to the requesting, requiring or purchasing of other information and does not use the genetic information for underwriting purposes.[63] The growing prevalence of genetic and genomic data in the medical record is likely to prompt more states to take steps to protect the citizen against genetic-based discrimination not only in health insurance but also other areas such as life insurance, employment, education, and housing. GINA has provided important protections, but these protections must be maintained and strengthened as large-scale genomic sequencing becomes more common and more accessible.

THE CURRENT
EVIDENCE SUPPORTING
PHARMACOGENETIC TESTING

There is mounting evidence showing a reduction in adverse drug reactions directly attributable to the regular use of pharmacogenetic testing in clinical practice. Almost all of the studies to date have shown improved clinical outcomes with appropriate use of this technology. Additionally, the evidence is quite compelling that the appropriate utilization of pharmacogenetic technology also reduces cost. It is the specialty of psychiatry that appears to hold the most promise for both.

> *Information dating back more than a decade indicates that psychiatric medications have been, for some time, among the most common medications found in patient deaths.*

Information dating back more than a decade indicates that psychiatric medications have been, for some time, among the most common medications found in patient deaths. A report published in 2005 by Drs. Paulozzi and Annest at the Centers for Disease Control (CDC) entitled Unintentional Poisoning Death: United States 1999 – 2004, found that opioids – 75.2 percent – were, by far, the most common medication associated with death by prescribed drugs during this period. The authors found the second most common prescribed medication to be benzodiazepines – at 29.4 percent – and the third to be antidepressants – at 17.6 percent.[64] The CDC's on-line *Drug Overdose in the United States: Fact Sheet* reports that in 2010 of the 38,329 drug overdose deaths in the US, 22,134 (sixty percent) of them were related to prescription drug overdoses. And of the 22,134 deaths, 6,497 (30 percent) involved benzodiazepines. In the CDC's same report, the authors note that in 2011 approximately 501,207 Emergency Department visits were related to anti-anxiety and insomnia medications.[65] [66] It is noteworthy to mention that all of the medications in the benzodiazepine family, and most of the medications in the sedative-hypnotic family are principally metabolized by the CYP450 enzyme system. In addition, polypharmacy carries a high risk of ADEs [67] as a result of drug-drug interactions (DDI) which are routinely evaluated in clinical practice. It remains, however, a formidable weakness in clinical practice that drug-gene interactions (DGI) and drug-drug-gene interactions (DDGI) are not routinely evaluated. An example of a common DDGI is a patient taking a drug that is metabolized by a particular CYP enzyme, is also taking a drug than is an inhibitor of that enzyme while simultaneously carrying a genetic variant in that same enzyme. These cumulative interactions can actually re-categorize patients from an intermediate metabolizer to a poor metabolizer of affected drugs and thus markedly increase the risk of suffering and ADE.[68]This problem is especially acute in elderly patients where polypharmacy is all too common and leads to higher risk of ADEs and higher incidence of treatment failure.[69] This problem also additionally results in higher healthcare resource utilization and costs. One way to reduce all three - ADEs, over-utilization and cost - is by routinely identifying DDIs, DGIs, and DDGIs in patients and modify drug regimens to prevent ADEs.

The New Mexico Psychiatric Pharmacogenetics Cohort Study was a study completed in June of 2013. It involved out-patient adult and adolescent (age > 15 y/o) psychiatric patients primarily of Caucasian, Hispanic and mixed-racial ethnicity. Using Genelex Corporation's proprietary risk analysis software, YouScript, as the database, patients were pre-screened for appropriateness of testing.[70] Genelex's YouScript Precision R$_x$ System is an algorithm driven genotyping method used to assist in the identification, diagnosis and treatment of patients at elevated risk of ADEs. It combines pharmacodynamic and pharmacokinetic interactions documented in clinical literature with a patented algorithm that mimics how the human body would metabolize multiple medications to predict changes in drug-levels and clinical effects. This allows YouScript to evaluate the combined effect of a patient's genetics and their entire drug regimen that considers cumulative drug and gene interactions where the magnitude of the increase or decrease in drug levels is often greater than any single interaction. Pharmacogenetic testing, based on medication regimen risk assessment, is of the 3 primary drug metabolizing enzymes from the CYP P450 family. The pre-screen criteria consisted of the aforementioned epidemiology and clinical utility of CYP2D6, CYP2C9 and CYP2C19 genotypes. Additionally, pre-screening criteria included patients with a history of several failed antidepressant/antipsychotic/psychotropic medication trials or a history of experiencing numerous side effects from these same classes of medications. Out of 348 patients, 296 were determined to meet criteria for pharmacogenetic testing. The results were impressive. In 82 of the patients, there was a revealed 101 previously unknown significant interaction risks (drug-drug/drug-gene interactions). Following pharmacogenetic testing the YouScript clinical decision support tool interprets test results, taking into account cumulative effects of medication regimen interactions and patient genetics, then suggests alternative, potentially safer treatments or other courses of action when advisable. Based on the results of pharmacogenetic testing, a major change in management occurred in 112 of the patients (38 percent). Utilizing the YouScript software to retrospectively analyze the potential for drug-drug/drug-gene interactions in the 296 patients, the power of predicting adverse interactions was shown to have markedly improved when compared to the trained clinician alone ($p < 0.005$). The software assigns one star as a mild to moderate risk of drug-drug/drug-gene interactions, two stars for a moderate risk of such interactions, and three stars for a high risk of drug-drug/drug-gene interactions. Of the 296 patients, 26 received a one star risk, 117 received a two star risk and 152 received a three star risk. Forty of the patients with a three star risk had no change to their treatment plan as their medication regimen did not warrant it. Utilization of the software, in addition to review by an experienced clinician, was evident to provide the greatest clinical utility. The combination of both was shown to be much more sensitive and specific ($p < 0.004$) in the process of pre-screening patients for pharmacogenetic testing. Thus, using a 'trained eye' in addition to drug-drug/drug-gene interaction prediction software was conclusively superior in reducing the risk of adverse drug reactions and improving treatment outcomes for patients than using either alone.[71]

In 2011 The Mayo Clinic completed a retrospective study of 60 outpatient adult psychiatric patients at the Hamm Clinic in St. Paul, Minnesota.[72] The results impressively showed a 31.2 percent reduction in depressive symptoms in those patients whose treatment was guided by pharmacogenetic testing compared to only a 7.2 percent reduction in depressive symptoms in those patients who were not tested (P < 0.02). A larger follow up replication study of 200 out-patient psychiatric patients by a Mayo Health System affiliate in La Cross, Wisconsin showed a 44.8 percent reduction in depressive symptoms in those patients whose treatment was guided by pharmacogenetic testing compared to a 26.4 percent reduction in those patients whose treatment was not guided by testing. This study yielded a much greater power in its results, with p < 0.001.[73][74]

> *...those who were slow-metabolizers in either the CYP2D6 or CYP2C19 enzymatic pathways had 69 percent more total health care visits, 67 percent more general medical visits, greater-than three-fold more medical absence days, and greater-than four-fold more disability claims.*

A more recent study by a research group at the University of Illinois, Department of Psychiatry completed in 2012 and published in 2013 employed a blinded retrospective method to follow 96 patients over one year. They utilized proprietary software by AssureRx to identify those patients at increased risk of adverse drug reactions, and found those who were slow-metabolizers in either the CYP2D6 or CYP2C19 enzymatic pathways had 69 percent more total health care visits, 67 percent more general medical visits, greater-than three-fold more medical absence days, and greater-than four-fold more disability claims.[75]

One of the more elegant studies was by Chou, et.al.[76] His team studied 100 psychiatric inpatient adults at Eastern State Hospital in Lexington, Kentucky. All patients were genotyped for CYP2D6 and individually tracked for adverse drug events (ADEs), hospital stays, and total costs over a 1-year period. The research team observed three dramatic trends. The first was a trend toward greater numbers of ADEs from psychotropic medications as one moved from patients with ultra-rapid CYP2D6 activity (UMs) to patients with absent CYP2D6 activity – poor metabolizers (PMs). The second trend was the average cost of treating patients with extremes in CYP2D6 activity (UM and PM) was $4,000 to $6,000 per year greater-than the cost of treating normal and intermediate metabolizers (IMs). The third trend was that CYP2D6 PMs had longer hospital stays. This study demonstrated that patients who are CYP2D6 poor metabolizers and CYP2D6 ultra-rapid metabolizers have more adverse drug events, longer hospital stays and simply cost more to treat. The proper application of pharmacogenetic technology is both a simple and precise answer to help reduce ADEs, reduce cost and better manage hospital stays.

> *This study demonstrated that patients who are CYP2D6 poor metabolizers and CYP2D6 ultra-rapid metabolizers have more adverse drug events, longer hospital stays and simply cost more to treat.*

A study published in 2013 by Ruano, Szarek, et.al. analyzed polymorphisms in CYP2D6 and length of stay in one-hundred fifty hospitalized subjects suffering from major depression at the Hartford Hospital Institute of Living. Although not a large study, it addressed the pervasive challenge of healthcare utilization. Just as Chou and his colleagues showed thirteen years earlier, Ruano and his team showed that those subjects who were CYP2D6 rapid or poor metabolizers had longer length of hospital stays. It further determined that CYP2D6 poor metabolizers had the most utilization of healthcare resources and the longest mean stays – 7.8 days compared to normal metabolizers (reference) at 5.7 days (p = 0.002).[77] Utilizing a Markov-based Monte Carlo microsimulation model to represent ADR events in the lifetime of a patient, Alagoz, Durham and Kasirajan illustrated that one-time pharmacogenetic testing was cost effective - via Incremental Cost-Effectiveness Ratio - by $43,165 per additional life-year and $53,680 per additional Quality-Adjusted Life Year.[78]

A 2013 study by Winner and Allen, et. al. found that pharmacogenetic testing strongly correlates with health resource utilization in psychiatric populations. They found that patients on a medication that has a high risk of adverse interactions with CYP450 genes (CYP2D6, CYP2C9, CYP2C19 and CYP1A2) or serotonin genes (SLC6A4 and 5HTR2A) were found to have 69% more healthcare visits and 67% more psychiatry visits compared to patients on medications not known to have significant drug-gene interactions.[79] Another study investigated the use of pharmacogenetics to guide the prescribing of psychotropic medications compared to standard therapy in patients with Major Depressive Disorder. The authors found an improvement in the pharmacogenetic guided group for all three depression scales used at 8 weeks for response rates (HAMD-17, p =0.03; QIDS-C16, p=0.005; and PHQ-9,p=0.01) and for remission (QIDS-16, p=0.03). In addition, they found that patients in the unguided group prescribed a medication discordant with their genotype experienced the least improvement (HAMD-17, p=0.007) and the patients in the guided group prescribed a medication concordant with their genotype showed the greatest improvement (HAMD-17, p=0.01).[80] In 200 subjects, the authors found a 44.8% reduction in depressive symptoms in patients who received treatment guided by pharmacogenetic testing compared to only 26.4% reduction in symptoms in those without testing.

The evidence supporting the use of pharmacogenetic technology is gaining momentum, not only for its utility in reducing drug-drug/drug-gene interactions, but as a tool to improve cost effectiveness. University of Utah researchers recently highlighted the impact of pharmacogenetic testing in elderly patients on healthcare costs at 4 months follow-up. Their cohort study compared 205 patients (age ≥65 years, taking ≥3 prescription medications and on ≥1 drugs metabolized by a polymorphic drug metabolizing enzymes) receiving pharmacogenetic testing (CYP2D6, CYP2C9, CYP2C19, CYP3A4, CYP3A5 & VKORC1) via Genelex Corporation's YouScript Personalized Prescribing System to 820 historical control patients who did not have pharmacogenetic testing. They found that among the tested group, there was a 39% decrease in the number of hospitalized patients (p=0.02) and a 71% reduction in ER visits (p=0.0002). This study elegantly showed that targeted pharmacogenetic testing resulted in health resource utilization (HRU) - related net cost savings of $218/patient compared to the untested group, including the COST of the CDST recommendations. Most of the providers who utilized the test (95 percent) considered the test helpful and nearly half (46 percent) followed CDST recommendations.[81] [82] The study team focused on four key areas that showed a variance of statistical trend relative to the results of pharmacogenetic testing interpreted via YouScript: patient test sample size, assessment of length of hospital stay, race stratification, and costs associated from administrative claims. By following the predictive value of this information, there was a 76% reduction in ER visits (p=0.0001), and a 21% decrease in the number of outpatient visits (p=0.0001). Potential mean cost savings in the tested group was estimated at $1,312 per patient. [83] These results were consistent with the previously published interim analysis results demonstrating that pharmacogenetic testing for drug metabolizing enzymes of the elderly exposed to polypharmacy, along with appropriate clinical decision support tools may result in lower HRU utilization and lower costs. These studies clearly illustrated the value of pharmacogenetic testing in the elderly population not only from a clinical value, but as a metric to control health resource utilization and costs. Elderly patients can realize a greater benefit from genetic testing as they are at higher risk for polypharmacy, adverse drug events, health utilization and overall costs.

SUBSTRATES, INHIBITORS, INDUCERS AND THE DRUG-PROTEIN COMPLEX

Numerous medications, nutrients, and herbal supplements are metabolized through the cytochrome P450 system. They can be inhibited or induced by drugs and, once altered, can be clinically significant in the development of drug-drug interactions that may cause unanticipated adverse reactions or therapeutic failures. Drugs that cause CYP450 drug interactions are referred to as either inhibitors or inducers.

Substrate: A chemical agent – a drug – that is metabolized by an enzyme into a metabolic end product. This generally results in the deactivation of the drug in the process of preparing it for elimination from the body. Prodrugs, however, are inactive drugs that must first be activated via metabolism. Thus, enzymes metabolize prodrugs into active compounds.

Inhibitor: A chemical agent that interferes with the function of an enzyme that metabolizes a given substrate. Enzymatic inhibition occurs in two different ways. The first – *competitive inhibition* – occurs when two substrates compete for the same binding site on an enzyme. One of the two substrates binds much more tightly to the enzyme and, thus, effectively displaces or disallows the other substrate from binding.

The active drug of the displaced substrate can then accumulate in the blood and become toxic. The second type of inhibition – *noncompetitive or allosteric inhibition* –occurs when a drug binds to a different site on an enzyme than that of a substrate. The enzyme becomes rather burdened and does not function as efficiently. The substrate(s) of this enzyme are then metabolized less efficiently and can accumulate in the blood, leading to increased risk of toxicity. Take, for example, Abilify (Aripiprazole). It is a substrate of CYP2D6, and predominantly metabolized by this enzyme. Let's say a patient is on an antipsychotic dose, perhaps 20mg at bedtime, but is becoming rather depressed. He is started on Cymbalta (Duloxetine) to treat his symptoms. Now, Duloxetine is also a substrate of CYP2D6 and is predominantly metabolized by this enzyme. Both Aripriprazole and Duloxetine can act as inhibitors, and tie up the CYP2D6 enzyme, however;

Duloxetine is a much stronger inhibitor. As Duloxetine is titrated from 30mg q/day to 60mg q/day, Aripriprazole serum levels increase as the CYP2D6 enzyme is saturated and has increasingly reduced ability to metabolize Aripiprazole. Thus, the risk of adverse effects from this medication – such as akathisia, dyskinesia and abnormal involuntary movements – is substantially increased. If Duloxetine was felt to be an ideal clinical choice for treatment, the dose should be started at the lowest possible – 20mg q/day – and the patient should be observed very carefully for any adverse effects. Additionally, serum Aripiprazole and its active metabolite, dehydroaripiprazole, should be monitored.

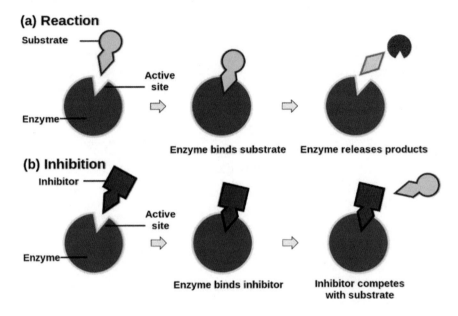

(a) Reaction

Substrate

Active site

Enzyme

Enzyme binds substrate   Enzyme releases products

(b) Inhibition

Inhibitor

Active site

Enzyme

Enzyme binds inhibitor   Inhibitor competes with substrate

<u>Inducer</u>: A chemical agent that increases the production of a particular enzyme. Substrates that are metabolized by this enzyme are metabolized at an increased rate. In a state of enzymatic induction, there are more intermediate metabolites present and more rapid depletion of a substrate. Simply put, there are more active enzymes present which work to breakdown a drug at a higher rate. Take, for example, Amitriptyline. It is a principal substrate of CYP2C19 and, to a lesser extent, CYP2D6 and, to a much lesser extent, CYP1A2. Both St. John's Wort and Ginkgo Biloba are inducers of CYP2C19. Thus, if a patient is taking these common supplements, there will be an increase in the amount of CYP2C19 enzymes

in the liver and gut. The metabolization of Amitriptyline will be increased - thus decreasing blood Amitriptyline levels – yielding increased blood levels of its secondary active metabolite Nortriptyline. Nortriptyline is also a principal substrate of CYP2C19 and CYP2D6. If CYP2D6 becomes saturated, the acting 'back-up' enzyme CYP3A4 then takes over the metabolization of Nortriptyline.[84]

Some of the CYP450 inducers and inhibitors are commonly ingested items such as grapefruit juice and tobacco. In the case of grapefruit juice, there are numerous medications known to interact with grapefruit juice including statins, antiarrhythmic agents, immunosuppressive agents, and calcium channel blockers. Since the inhibition of the enzyme system seems to be dose dependent, the more a patient drinks, the stronger the enzyme inhibition. Additionally, the effects can last for several days if grapefruit juice is consumed on a regular basis.

Drug-Protein Complex: Proteins are the vehicles which carry drugs in the bloodstream. Some drugs are highly protein bound and some are poorly protein bound. It is important to look at patients' protein status when prescribing drugs. Low protein levels most certainly can increase free drug levels in the blood and thereby substantially increase the risk of toxicity and drug-drug interactions. Take Depakote (Valproic Acid) for example. The plasma binding protein of Depakote is dependent on its dose (concentration in the blood). At approximately 40 mcg/mL about 90 percent of Depakote is bound to protein and, thus, inactive and about 10 percent of the drug being free and, thus, active. When, however, plasma concentrations increase to approximately 130 mcg/mL then free, active, Depakote levels increase to approximately 19 percent. As with most drugs, even higher than expected free fractions occur in the elderly, as protein production and regulation becomes less efficient as we age. Additionally, protein dysregulation is also higher in prevalence in patients with hepatic and renal disease and in patients with hyperlipidemia. Most patients in contemporary psychiatry are on a myriad of medications from a number of prescribers. Many of these drugs compete for proteins. Whenever possible, it makes far more clinical sense to order free medication levels as they reflect the unbound – active portion – of the drug.

In 2015, we completed one of the largest retrospective studies examining the frequency of complex pharmacokinetic-pharmacodynamic interactions. The study consisted of more than 20,000 patients who had been referred for pharmacogenetic testing. The enzymes CYP2D6, CYP2C9, CYP2C19, CYP3A4 and CYP3A5 were analyzed for interaction type. This study examined the frequency of drug-drug interaction (DDI), drug-gene interaction (DGI) and drug-drug-gene interaction (DDGI). The study's major finding was that DGIs and DDGIs represented 25 percent and 22 percent respectively of the total interactions observed.[85] The study clearly showed that the older – Medicare – cohort was at increased risk for these cumulative interactions due to increased polypharmacy. These studies highlight the prevalence of genetic risk for out of range drug levels in polypharmacy-treated patients as a consequence of the low incidence of normal metabolizers. Many previous studies have shown that more than 75 percent of patients [86] have variations in at least one CYP enzyme, and may not respond to medications the way a prescriber expects.

The chart below shows the frequency of drug-drug interaction (DDI), drug-gene interaction (DGI) and drug-drug-gene interaction (DDGI).

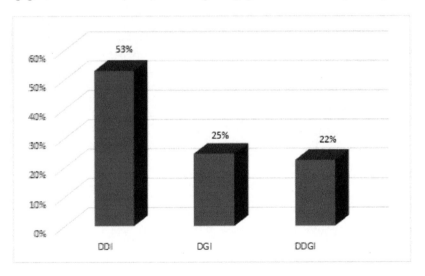

EPIDEMIOLOGY AND CLINICAL UTILITY OF THE CYP2D6 ENZYME

The CYP2D6 gene is located on chromosome 22. The CYP2D6 enzyme processes many common medications, including opioid analgesics, antipsychotics, antidepressants and chemotherapeutics. For psychiatry, this enzyme is, by far, the most important CYP enzyme tested in clinical practice because approximately 85 percent of antidepressant medications and 40 percent of antipsychotic medications are either predominantly or substantially metabolized by it.

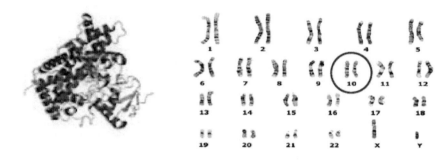

Structure of
CYP 2C19 Enzyme

Ploidy of Human Chromosomes (male)
with Chromosome 10 circled

Approximately 35 percent of the population has a non-functional CYP2D6 allele, which substantially increases the risk of adverse drug reactions with patients who are taking multiple medications. Approximately 8 percent of Caucasians and US Latinos are Poor Metabolizers. CYP2D6 Poor Metabolizer patients carry two loss-of-function alleles. These patients will require substantially lower doses of a drug and have high risk of adverse drug effects which can produce physiologic toxicity quickly. Approximately 35 percent of Caucasians and US Latinos are Intermediate Metabolizers (IMs). CYP2D6 Intermediate Metabolizers received one normal functioning allele and one loss-of-function allele from each parent respectively. The loss-of-function of IMs vary from about 20 to 70 percent, so an IM patient's clinical history of response to psychotropic medications and how their first-degree relatives have responded to psychotropic medications hold the greatest weight in forming a prognosis of how a given IM patient will respond.

Patients who are CYP2D6 Ultra-Rapid Metabolizers carry more than two copies of functional alleles. Comparatively, individuals of Arabic / Mediterranean ethnicity seem to have a higher prevalence of UM polymorphisms in the CYP2D6 enzyme.[87] Almost all patients who are UMs will give a history of having almost no response to medications that are predominantly metabolized by the CYP2D6 pathway. Clinicians will often hear things like "I ate them like candy and they didn't do anything", or "None of those drugs did anything at all". Patients who are UMs will most often require 50 percent to 100 percent more medication to have a clinical response.

> *For psychiatry, this enzyme is, by far, the most important CYP enzyme tested in clinical practice because approximately 85 percent of antidepressant medications and 40 percent of antipsychotic medications are either predominantly or substantially metabolized by this enzyme.*

Approximately 25 percent of Asians are estimated to be CYP2D6 poor metabolizers (PMs). Asian ultra-rapid metabolizers (UMs) range from 0 to 2 percent (CYP2D6 UMs are estimated at 1 percent or less). It is evident from the high prevalence of CYP2D6 poor and intermediate metabolizers in Asians that ordering CYP2D6 genotyping and phenotyping for an Asian patient is clinically useful for those patients who have a history of experiencing side effects with CYP2D6 substrates or at higher risk of drug-drug interactions – such as the elderly. Ordering CYP2D6 phenotyping and genotyping for African-Americans is only slightly more useful. Albeit they have a similar low prevalence of PMs and UMs as do Asians – with approximately one percent of African Americans being PMs and two percent being UMs – they have the largest population of IMs at approximately 40 to 50 percent.[88]

This CYP2D6 enzyme is a high affinity, low capacity enzyme. If a patient is a CYP2D6 poor-metabolizer, as the concentration of the drug or drugs they are taking increase, this enzyme will be quickly saturated and metabolism will spill over into the CYP3A4 and CYP1A2 enzymatic pathways. Both of these pathways are low-affinity, high capacity pathways and weakly bind larger amounts of drug. One can see that there remains substantial room for drugs that utilize the CYP2D6 pathway to become toxic. Thus, pharmacogenetic testing should be ordered for Caucasian, Latin-American, or African American patients who are being prescribed numerous medications which utilize the CYP2D6 pathway, have a history of failing numerous psychotropic medications, or who have a history of experiencing numerous adverse drug reactions.

Common CYP2D6 substrates in the psychotropic class are numerous and include Amitriptyline (co-metabolized by CYP2C19), Doxepin (co-metabolized by CYP2C19), Imipramine (co-metabolized with CYP1A2), Nortriptyline, Fluvoxamine (co-metabolized by CYP1A2), Fluoxetine (co-metabolized to a minor extent by CYP3A4), Paroxetine, Venlafaxine, Duloxetine, Trazodone, Bupropion, Perphenazine, Haloperidol, Aripiprazole, Risperidone, Atomoxetine (Strattera), Dextroamphetamine (Dexedrine), Hydroxyzine, Promethazine, and Buspirone.

For the psychiatric clinician, it is also important to take note that the CYP2D6 enzyme also primarily metabolizes Codeine, Oxycodone, Hydrocodone and Tramadol. The number of cases of patients – especially the elderly – suffering from adverse medication effects and overdoses from these medications is extraordinary. In his book, Dr. David Mzarek emphasizes the importance of the relationship with CYP2D6 polymorphisms to suicidality and activation of a manic episode in bipolar illness:

> *"Two additional considerations further justify the identification of patients with the poor metabolizer phenotype when using SSRIs that are CYP2D6 substrate medications. The first is that such patients may be more likely to develop suicidal ideation during the first weeks of treatment with CYP2D6 substrate medications because of a rapid rise in serum level of these medications. The second consideration is that patients with the poor CYP2D6 metabolizer phenotype who have a genetic vulnerability to develop bipolar disorder may be more likely to have an activation of a manic episode if treated with an SSRI that is a CYP2D6 substrate medication at standard dose."* [89]

Medications Metabolized by CYP2D6 (Substrates)
*medications of most importance to psychiatry are in blue

Atomoxetine (Strattera)	Nortryptiline (Pamelor)
Bufuralol	Ondansetron (Zofran)
Carvedilol (Coreg)	Oxycodone
Chlorpropamide	Palonoetron (Aloxil)
Clorpromazine (Thorazine)	Paroxetine (Paxil)
Clomipramine (Anafranil)	Perhexiline (Pexid)
Clonidine (Catapres)	Phenacetin
Clozapine	Phenformin
Codeine	Perphenazine
Debrisoquine	Promethazine (Phenergen)
Desipramine (Norparmin)	Propafenone (Rythmol)
Desmethylcitalopram	Propanololol (Inderal)
Dextromethorphan	Protryptiline (Vivactil)
Diphenhydramine (Benadryl)	Risperidone (Risperdal)
Dolasetron (Anzemet)	Tamoxifen (Nolvadex)
Donepezil (Aricept)	Thioridazine (Mellaril)
Doxepin (Sinequan)	Timolol (Blocadren)
Duloxetine (Cymbalta)	Tolterodine (Detrol)
Encainide (Enkaid)	Tramadol (Ultram)
Flecanide (Tambocor)	Trazodone (Desyrel)
Fluoxetine (Prozac)	Venlafaxine (Effexor)
Fluvoxamine (Luvox)	Zuclopenthixol
Haldoperidol (Haldol)	
Hydrocodone (Vicodin)	
Imipramine (Tofranil)	

Medications that Inhibit CYP2D6 (Inhibitors)
*medications of most importance to psychiatry are in blue

Amiodarone (Cordarone)
Buproprion (Wellbutrin)
Cimetidine
Chloroquine (Aralen)
Cinacalcet (Sensipar)
Diphenhydramine (Benadryl)
Duloxetine (Cymbalta)
Fluoxetine (Prozac)
Haldoperidol (Haldol)

Imatinib (Gleevec)
Methadone
Paroxetine (Paxil)
Propafenone (Rhythmol)
Propoxyphene (Darvon)
Quinidine (Quinidex)
Sertraline (Zoloft)
Terbinafine (Lamisil)
Thioridazine (Mellaril)

The table below gives examples of specific dose adjustments of antidepressants and antipsychotics based on CYP2D6-mediated influence[90] along with characteristics for different CYP2D6 phenotypes.[91] The table adapted from information in Kirchheiner's review article[92] includes several similar tables and charts based on CYP2D6 status.

Characteristics	Poor Metabolizers	Intermediate Metabolizers	Extensive Metabolizers	Ultra-rapid metabolizers
Major variants	CYP2D6 *3, *4,*5,*6	CYP2D6 *9, *10,*41	CYP2D6 *1	Multiple copies of CYP2D6
Enzyme activity	Inactive	Low residual	Normal	Very high
Plasma drug level	High			Very low
Clinical consequence	Risk of drug-related side effects			Loss of drug efficacy
Dose	Use of reduced drug dose	Lower dose for some patients	Standard dose for most patients	Higher drug dose required

Drugs	Poor Metabolizers	Intermediate Metabolizers	Extensive Metabolizers	Ultra-rapid metabolizers
	Percent of Standard Dose			
Imipramine (Tofranil)	30	80	130	180
Doxepin (Sinequan)	35	80	130	175
Trimipramine (Surmontil)	35	90	130	180
Despramine (Norpramin)	40	80	125	170
Nortriptyline (Pamelor)	55	95	120	150
Clomipramine (Anafranil)	60	90	110	145
Paroxetine (Paxil)	65	85	115	135
Venlafaxine (Effexor)	70	80	105	130
Amitriptyline (Elavil)	75	90	105	130
Bupropion (Wellbutrin)	90	95	105	110
Perphenazine (Trilafon)	30	80	125	175
Haloperidol (Haldol)	75	95	100	115
Olanzapine (Zyprexa)	60	105	120	150
Risperidone (Risperdal)	85	90	100	110

Dose-adjustment values were determined by comparing drug concentration, clearance, or exposure data across phenotypes. Values have been approximated by the authors to the nearest 5 percent.[93]

A variety of nomenclature systems have been developed to describe allele variation and haplotypes of ADME (Absorption, Distribution, Metabolism, and Excretion) genes.[94] The most common is the "star" (*) system and has been widely adopted in the field. In most cases, *1 stand for the default reference (wild type or fully functional) allele or haplotype, while other designations (e.g. *2 or *3 etc.) define haplotypes carrying one or more genetic variants.[95] The *1 allele definition is usually based on the subpopulation in which the gene was initially studied, and may not necessarily indicate the most common allele in all populations. In few cases, *1 is not the reference allele; for example, *NAT2*4* is the reference allele for the *NAT2* gene as it is the most common functional allele across human populations.[96] Clinical laboratories report a variant of one or more allele-defining sequence variations are found and in their absence default to a reference allele (often *1) assignment. Therefore, such reference allele (*1) designation is assigned contingent on which variants were assayed, but does not consider variants not included in the assay (i.e., an assigned *1 carrier may still have genetic variants that the test was not designed to detect). In other words, a negative result for the alleles tested by the assay (and the assignment of the *1 reference allele) does not eliminate the possibility that other non-functional alleles may be present.[97] The lists of haplotypes and nomenclature for pharmacogenetic genes can be found on a variety of gene or gene family specific websites that are usually maintained by specific nomenclature committees. For example, Human Cytochrome P450 (CYP) Allele Nomenclature Database[98] and SuperCYP[99] are two such reference websites. The information about pharmacogenetics haplotypes is also available through more comprehensive sites, such as the Pharmacogenomics Knowledge Base.[100]

The table below shows CYP2D6 frequency for some significant alleles.[101][102][103][104][105][106] Other or rarer variants are not included due to variance in frequencies and/or unknown clinical significance.

Allele	Enzyme Activity	Ethnic Background			
		Caucasian	African American	East Asian	Middle Eastern
*2	Functional	26.9%	14.2%	12.8%	21.7%
*3	Non-functional	1.3%	0.3%	0.0%	0.1%
*4	Non-functional	18.5%	6.2%	0.4%	7.8%
*5	Non-functional	2.7%	6.1%	5.6%	2.3%
*6	Non-functional	1%	0.2%	0%	0.7%
*9	Reduced-function	2.1%	0.5%	0.1%	0%
*10	Reduced-function	3.2%	4.2%	42.3%	3.5%
*17	Reduced-function	0.3%	18.2%	0%	1.6%
*41	Reduced-function	8.6%	9.4%	2%	20.4%

We recently completed a retrospective analysis on 22,225 patients (7.5 percent of the referrals were from psychiatry) who had been referred for pharmacogenetic testing of CYP2D6. We examined the frequency of CYP2D6 metabolic phenotypes. The CYP2D6 variants tested included: *2, *2A, *3 -*12, *14A, *15, *17, *19, *20, *29, *36, *41, and gene duplications. We found that nearly half of the subjects – 7.1 percent – evaluated for CYP2D6 were categorized as either intermediate metabolizers, poor metabolizers or ultra-rapid metabolizers.

The tested CYP2D6 phenotypic frequency of the mixed-race, U.S. based patients is shown below.[107]

CYP2D6 Phenotype	Prevalence
Normal Metabolizer	52.8%
Intermediate Metabolizer	37.7%
Poor Metabolizer	6.8%
Ultra Rapid Metabolizer	2.7%

EPIDEMIOLOGY AND CLINICAL UTILITY OF THE CYP2C19 ENZYME

The CYP2C19 gene is located on the long (q) arm of chromosome 10. Inheritance is autosomal recessive. The CYP2C19 enzyme metabolizes from 5-10 percent of prescribed drugs such as Clopidogrel, proton pump inhibitors, anticonvulsants, [108] [109] but approximately 38 percent of all antidepressant medications. Approximately 5 percent of Caucasians, 15 to 20 percent of Japanese and 12 to 20 percent of Africans have a slow acting, poor-metabolizer form of this drug metabolizing enzyme. [110] [111] Research to date indicates that there remains significant variability among populations. Probably the best example of this are Polynesians. The number of CYP2C19 Poor Metabolizers in Polynesians ranges widely from 38 to 79 percent depending on location. [112] [113] Thus the risk for variant alleles of CYP2C19 varies widely by ethnicity, with patients of East Asian ancestry having higher prevalence. [114] Multiple CYP2C19 SNPs associated with drug metabolism have been identified, with CYP2C19*2, *3 and *17 being the most significant. [115]

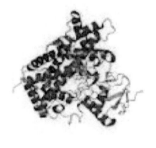

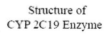

Structure of
CYP 2C19 Enzyme

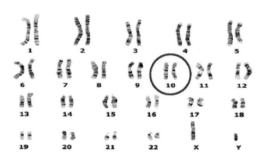

Ploidy of Human Chromosomes (male)
with Chromosome 10 circled

The CYP2C19*17 allele is associated with increased enzymatic activity. The data thus far has shown that ultra-rapid metabolizing CYP2C19*17 function in patients with this allele is only likely to be relevant if drugs with very narrow therapeutic windows are prescribed. Clopidogrel is probably the best known CYP2C19 substrate in the greater medical community. For psychiatric clinicians, however, since about 38 percent of antidepressants utilize CYP2C19 in some fashion – either predominantly or secondarily – it is very relevant. Although the poor metabolizer phenotype holds the greatest clinical significance at present, there is data that shows the incidence of adverse drug events relating to the CYP2C19 pathway is probably greater than estimated.[116] Common CYP2C19 substrates in the psychotropic class include Amitryptiline (co-metabolized by CYP2D6), Doxepin (co-metabolized by CYP2D6), Impramine, Citalopram, Escitalopram, Fluoxetine (co-metabolized by CYP2D6) Sertraline, and Diazepam. It is also important to note that the CYP2C19 enzyme primarily metabolizes Carisoprodol (Soma) – one of the more common drugs associated with abuse and overdoses.

Medications Metabolized by CYP2C19 (Substrates)
*medications of most importance to psychiatry are in blue

Aripiprazole (Abilify)
Amitryptiliine (Elavil)
Carisoprodol (Soma)
Citalopram (Celexa)
Clomipramine (Anafranil)
Clopidogrel (Plavix)
Cyclophosphamide (Endoxan)
Desipramine (Norpramin)
Diazepam (Valium)
Diphenhydramine (Benadryl)
Doxepin (Sinequan)
Escitalopram (Lexapro)
Fluoxetine (Prozac)
Imipramine (Tofranil)
Indomethacin
Labetolol (Trandate)
Lansoprazole (Prevacid)
Methadone

Mephenytoin (Mesantoin)
Moclobemide (Manerix)
Nelfinavir (Viracept)
Nilutamide (Anadron)
Olanzapine (Zyprexa)
Omeprazole (Prilosec)
Pantoprazole (Protonix)
Pentamidine
Phenobarbital
Phenytoin (Dilantin)
Proguanil
Propanolol (Inderal)
Rabeprazole (Aciphex)
Sertraline (Zoloft)
Thalidomide
Voriconazole

Medications that Inhibit CYP2C19 (Inhibitors)
*medications of most importance to psychiatry are in blue

Chloramphenicol
Cimetidine (Tagamet)
Clopidogrel (Plavix)
Delavirdine (Rescriptor)
Efavirez (Sustiva)
Esomeprazole (Nexium)
Felbamate (Felbatol)
Fluconazole (Diflucan)
Fluoxetine (Prozac)
Fluvoxamine (Luvox)

Isoniazid (Hydra)
Ketoconazole
Moclobemide (Manerix)
Modafinil (Provigil)
Omeprazole (Prilosec)
Oxcarbazepine (Trileptal)
Ticlopidine (Ticlid)
Probenecid (Probalan)
Topiramate (Topamax)
Voriconazole (Vfend)

Medications that Induce CYP2C19 (Inducers)
medications of most importance to psychiatry are in blue

Amioglutethimide
Artemisin
Barbiturates
Carbamazepine (Tegretol)
Efavirenz (Sustiva)
Phenytoin (Dilantin)

Primidone
Prednisone
Rifampin (Rifadin)
Rifapentine
Ritonavir (Norvir)
St. Johns wort

The table below shows CYP2C19 frequency for some significant alleles. Other, or rarer variants, are not included due to variance in frequencies and/or unknown clinical significance. [117] [118] [119] [120] [121]

Alleles	Enzyme Activity	Ethnic Background		
		Caucasian	African American	Asian
*1/*1	Two functional alleles	31%	29%	32%
*1/*2 or *1/*3	One loss-of-function and one functional allele	26%	29%	50%
*2/*2, *2/*3, *3/*3	Two loss-of-function alleles	2%	4%	14%
*1/*17, *17/*17	One or two gain-of-function alleles	41%	38%	4%

In our recent pharmacogenetics analysis of 22,225 patients, we also examined the frequency of CYP2C19 metabolic phenotypes. The CYP2C19 variants tested included: *2, *10, *12, *17. Our results showed that 57.9 percent of the subjects evaluated for CYP2C19 were categorized as either intermediate metabolizers, poor metabolizers or ultra-rapid metabolizers.

The tested CYP2C19 phenotypic frequency of the mixed-race, U.S. based patients is shown below.[122]

CYP2C19 Phenotype	Prevalence
Normal Metabolizer	42.1%
Intermediate Metabolizer	25.8%
Poor Metabolizer	2.6%
Ultra Rapid Metabolizer	29.5%

EPIDEMIOLOGY AND CLINICAL UTILITY OF THE CYP2C9 ENZYME

The CYP2C9 enzyme metabolizes between 10 and 20 percent of all drugs including warfarin, phenytoin, non-steroidal anti-inflammatory drugs (NSAIDs), and antihyperglycemic sulphonylureas. [123] The CYP2C9 enzyme locus is also located on chromosome 10. It is the second most abundant cytochrome enzyme representing approximately 20 percent of CYP enzymes representing approximately 20 percent of CYP activity in the liver, and is responsible for metabolizing about 15 percent of drugs undergoing Phase I metabolism. [124] Approximately 10 percent of the total populations are poor metabolizers (PMs); however, approximately 35 percent of Caucasians are PMs. [125] [126] There is growing evidence that Japanese and Ethiopians have an increased prevalence of CYP2C9 polymorphisms and thus may have more poor metabolizers in their populations. [127] This enzyme is particularly susceptible to significant interactions because it plays a more prominent role in metabolizing medications with low therapeutic index – such as Dilantin (Phenytoin) and Phenobarbital. [128] Multiple SNPs have been identified that may be associated with drug metabolism, with the *2 and *3 variants being the most significant, leading to poor metabolism phenotypes. [129]

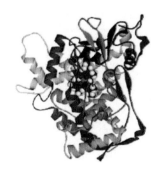

Structure of CYP2C9 Enzyme

There is a low threshold for toxicity in these medications. Individuals who are CYP2C9 PMs who are prescribed Phenytoin or Barbiturates should be prescribed 50 percent of the standard dose of these medications respectively. Barbiturates and carbamazepine are inducers of the CYP2C9 enzyme and can substantially increase its activity. Phenytoin (Dilantin) is a CYP2C9 substrate, inhibitor, and inducer. Clinically, however, adverse outcomes primarily have been due to Phenytoin's susceptibility to toxicity when combined with CYP2C9 inhibitors – Valproic Acid and Phenytoin are two such examples – and its ability to act as an inducer of CYP2C9 and other CYP450 enzymes, thus reducing the effect of many other medications.[130] Valproic Acid (Depakote) also has an inhibitory effect on CYP2C9 enzyme activity. Thus, if Depakote is given with other medications that are primarily metabolized by the CYP2C9 pathway – such as Phenytoin – the blood levels of that medication can become toxic.[131]

This enzyme is particularly susceptible to significant interactions because it plays a more prominent role in metabolizing medications with low therapeutic index – such as Dilantin (Phenytoin) and Phenobarbital.

Psychiatric clinicians should always remember that Depakote is very highly protein bound. In addition to enzyme inhibition, aspirin can displace Depakote and cause free levels to become toxic in some patients. There is also mounting evidence that patients who have a specific CYP2C9 genetic polymorphism – namely CYP2C9*2 and CYP2C9*3 – tend to biotransform Depakote (VPA) into its hepatotoxic metabolite, 4-ene-VPA. Thus, one should take great care with Depakote dosing in patients who possess these specific polymorphisms or who are poor CYP2C9 metabolizers.[132] Moreover, co-administration of medications that can reduce Glutathione levels, such as Acetaminophen, particularly increase an individual's susceptible to toxicity.

Medications Metabolized by CYP2C9 (Substrates)
*medications of most importance to psychiatry are in blue

Alosetron (Lotronex)
Bosentan (Tracleer)
Candesartan (Atacand)
Celecoxib (Celebrex)
Chlopropanide (Diabinese)
Diclofenac (Voltaren)
Dronabinol (Marinol)
Flurbiprofen (Ansaid)
Fluvastatin (Lescol)
Glimepiride (Amaryl)
Glipizide (Glucotrol)
Glyburide (DiaBeta)
Ibuprofen (Motrin, Advil)
Indomethacin (Indocin)
Irbesartan (Avapro)

Losartan (Cozaar)
Meloxicam (Mobic)
Montelukast (Singulair)
Naproxen (Aleve)
Nateglinide (Starlix)
Phenobarbital
Phenytoin (Dilantin)
Piroxicam (Feldene)
Rosiglitazone (Avandia)
Rosuvastatin (Crestor)
Sulfamethoxazole
Tolbutamide
Torsemide (Demadex)
Valsartan (Diovan)
Warfarin (Coumadin)

Medications that Inhibit CYP2C9 (Inhibitors)
*medications of most importance to psychiatry are in blue

Amiodarone (Cordarone)
Clopridogrel (Plavix)
Delavirdine (Rescriptor)
Disulfarim (Antabuse)
Doxifluridine
Efavirenz (Sustiva)
Fluconazole (Diflucan)
Fluorouracil (5-FU)
Imatinib (Gleevec)
Isoniazid (Hydra)
Leflunomide (Arava)

Metronidazole (Flagyl)
Miconazole (Monistat)
Paroxetine (Paxil)
Phenytoin (Dilantin)
Sertraline (Xoloft)
Sulfamethoxazole
Sulfaphenazone
Sulfinpyrazone
Valproic Acid (Depakote)
Voriconazole (Vfend)

Medications that Induce CYP2C9 (Inducers)
medications of most importance to psychiatry are in blue

Aminoglutethimide(Cytadren)
Barbiturates
Bosentan (Tracleer)
Carbamazepine (Tegretol)
Griseofulvin (Grifulvin V)
Nevirapine (Viramine)

Phenytoin (Dilantin)
Primidone
Rifabutin
Rifampin
Rifapentine (Priftin)
St. Johns Wort

The table below shows CYP2C9 frequency for some significant alleles. [133] Other or rarer variants are not included due to variance in frequencies and/or unknown clinical significance.

Allele	Enzyme Activity[1]	Ethnic Background			
		Caucasian	Asian	African American	Hispanic
*2	Decreased	15.1%	2.9%	2.8%	6.9%
*3	Decreased	5.7%	3.9%	2.0%	6.4%
*5	Decreased	-	-	1.5%	1.5%
*8	Decreased	-	1.0%	4.7%	1.5%
*11	Decreased	0.5%	-	1.3%	1.0%

We also completed pharmacogenetics analysis of the CYP2C9 enzymes on our subject population of 22,649 patients. We examined the frequency of CYP2C9 metabolic phenotypes. The CYP2C9 variants tested included: *2 -*6, *8, *11, *13, *15. Our results showed that 57.9 percent of the subjects evaluated for CYP2C9 were categorized as either intermediate metabolizers or poor metabolizers.

The tested CYP2C9 phenotypic frequency of the mixed-race, U.S. based patients is shown below.[135]

CYP2C9 Phenotype	Prevalence
Normal Metabolizer	67.5%
Intermediate Metabolizer	29.1%
Poor Metabolizer	3.4%

EPIDEMIOLOGY AND CLINICAL UTILITY OF THE CYP1A2 ENZYME

The CYP1A2 enzyme is responsible for the primary metabolization of approximately 5 to 10 percent of drugs in clinical use today. It is located on chromosome 15. Particularly important for psychiatry, it metabolizes Clozapine, Imipramine (co-metabolized by CYP2D6), Fluvoxamine (co-metabolized by CYP2D6) and caffeine. This enzyme often collects drugs that have bypassed CYP2D6 after it has been saturated. In contrast to CYP2D6, which is a high affinity - low capacity enzyme, the CYP1A2 enzyme is a high capacity - low affinity enzyme and thus can handle more volume of drug. CYP1A2 is of particular interest because of the unique CYP1A2 hyper-inducer phenotype. In the presence of one of these inducers such as carbamazepine, phenytoin or smoking the amount of CYP1A2 induction

Smoking induces ("speeds up") CYP1A2 causing it to more rapidly metabolizes other substrates (e.g. medications) which may be present.

has been shown to significantly increase relative to an individual without the hyperinducer phenotype. [136] Smoking induces ("speeds up") CYP1A2 causing it to more rapidly metabolize other substrates (e.g. medications) which may be present leading to a reduced therapeutic effect. Thus, as most schizophrenics are heavy smokers, they usually require an increased dose of Clozapine. Often, when they are hospitalized in a facility with a non-smoking policy – which today is most hospitals – they become over-sedated and have an increased risk of extrapyramidal side effects and blood dyscrasias if their dose is not adequately reduced. Patients of Japanese, Egyptian and Caucasian descent are particularly susceptible to hyper-induction. Thus, they will more than likely require the greatest increase in dose if they regularly use products that contain nicotine (e.g. cigarettes and oral tobacco products), and will require a respective reduction in dose when hospitalized.

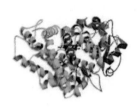

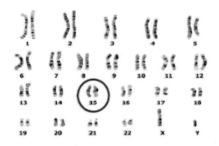

Structure of CYP1A2 Enzyme

Ploidy of Human Chromosomes (male)
with Chromosome 15 circled

Medications Metabolized by CYP1A2 (Substrates)
*medications of most importance to psychiatry are in blue

Amitryptiline (Elavil)
Alosetron (Lotronex)
Caffeine
Clomipramine (Anafranil)
Clozapine (Clozaril)
Cyclobenzaprine
Duloxetine
Estradiol
Flutamide (Eulexin)
Frovatriptan (Frova)
Fluvoxamine (Luvox)
Haldoperidol (Haldol)
Imipramine
Melatonin
Mexiletine (Mexitil)
Mirtazepine (Remeron)
Naproxen

Odansatron (Zofran)
Olanzapine (Zyprexa)
Propanolol (Inderal)
Ramelteon (Rozerem)
Ropinrole (Requip)
Tacrine (Cognex)
Theophyline
Tizanidine (Zanaflex)
Triamterene (Dyrenium)
Verapamil
Zolmitriptan (Zomig)

Medications that Inhibit CYP1A2 (Inhibitors)
*medications of most importance to psychiatry are in blue

Amiodarone
Artemisinin
Atazanavir (Reyataz)
Cimedidine (Tagamet)
Cimetidine (Tagamet)
Ciprofoxacin (Cipro)
Efavirenz
Enoxacin

Estradiol
Fluoroquinolones
Fluvoxamine (Luvox)
Interferon
Mexiletine (Mexitil)
Tacrine (Cognex)
Ticopidine
Thiabendazole
Zileuton (Zyflo)

Medications/Substances that Induce CYP1A2 (Inducers)
*medications of most importance to psychiatry are in blue

Barbiturates
Cruciferous vegetables
Nitrates from grilled meat
Carbamazepine (Tegreol)
Omeprazole
Primidone
Rifampin (Rifadin)
Smoking

The table below shows the allele frequency of CYP1A2*1F.[137] Other or rarer variants are not in included due to variance in frequencies and/or unknown clinical significance.

Allele	Enzyme Activity	Ethnic Background			
		Caucasian	Asian	African American	Hispanic
*1F	Higher Inducibility	32-58%	8-37%	40-51%	32%

EPIDEMIOLOGY AND CLINICAL UTILITY OF THE CYP3A4 / 3A5 ENZYMES

The CYP3A isoenzymes make up the largest family of CYP450 proteins in the liver.[138] The CYP3A4 enzyme is the most abundant P450 enzyme in the liver, accounting for about 30 percent of all P450 enzyme content in this organ. The CYP3A4 / 3A5 enzymes are involved, in one way or another, in the metabolization of approximately fifty percent of all prescribed medications. They are, however, rarely the predominant players.[139] The loci for both enzymes are located on chromosome 7. These enzymes are high capacity - low affinity enzymes. They are non-specific and most often work as a team when metabolizing a drug.[140] Important to psychiatry, these enzymes are significantly involved in metabolizing Alprazolam, Clonazepam (also metabolized by the NAT2 pathway), Diazepam (co-metabolized by CYP2C19), Midazolam, Triazolam, Buspirone (co-metabolized with CYP2D6), Haldol, Propranolol (co-metabolized with CYP2D6), Trazodone (co-metabolized with CYP2D6), Fluvoxamine (co-metabolized with CYP2D6), Nefazodone, Norfluoxetine (after Fluoxetine is first metabolized by CYP2D6), Carbamazepine, Topiramate, Modafinil, Ziprasidone (after co-metabolized by primary CYP2D6), Zolpidem, and Zaleplon. Additionally, these enzymes primarily metabolize St. Jonh's Wort, Cocaine, and Dextromethorphan. The CYP3A4 / 3A5 enzymes are essentially the backup metabolizer team to their CYP2D6 cousin.

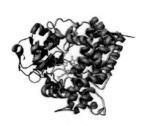

Structure of CYP 3A4 Enzyme

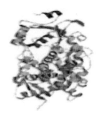

Structure of CYP 3A5 Enzyme

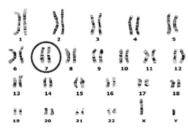

Ploidy of Human Chromosomes (male) with Chromosome 7 circled

It is important to reiterate that CYP2D6 is a high affinity, low capacity enzyme, whereas the CYP3A4 / 3A5 enzymes are low affinity but high capacity. When CYP2D6 becomes saturated, the spillover of excess drug falls to the CYP3A4 / 3A5 enzymes. Despite their role as 'secondary players', the CYP3A enzyme class is no less important as it comprises approximately 82 percent of CYP450 enzyme content in the human intestine.[141]

> *The CYP3A4 / 3A5 enzymes are essentially the backup metabolizer team to their 2D6 cousin.*

The CYP3A4 enzyme is unique among the cytochromes because it has multiple substrate binding sites, which is the likely reason it can metabolize so many drugs.[142] There are reports of 10- to 100-fold or more variation in CYP3A4 liver expression across the population, but single nucleotide polymorphisms have been unable to explain the highly variable enzymatic activity of the encoded protein.[143][144] Interestingly, studies have shown women have up to 25 percent higher CYP3A4 activity than men.[145] Thus it is likely that the high variation results from a combination of age, gender, genetics, and environmental influences.[146][147]

The epidemiology of these enzymes is not as robust as that of the CYP2D6, CYP2C19, CYP2C9 and CYP1A2 enzymes. Polymorphisms of the CYP3A4 enzyme across all ethnicities occur at a frequency of less-than five percent. Until recently, the clinical utility of known CYP3A4 variants was questionable. However, in 2011, a new variant allele, CYP3A4*22, was discovered. It influences hepatic expression of CYP3A4 and response to statin drugs.[148][149] It could also serve as a biomarker for the CYP3A4 metabolizer phenotype.

There is a high degree of sequence homology between CYP3A4 and CYP3A5, and thus there is an overlap of substrates. Both first-pass metabolism and systemic clearance of drugs metabolized by CYP3A5 are susceptible to genetically determined differences in enzyme expression.[150] Polymorphisms in CYP3A5 may be significant for a number of commonly prescribed medications across multiple specialties. The variant alleles for CYP3A5 may result in truncated mRNA with loss of expression of the functional protein. The prevalence of CYP3A5 variants differs widely by ethnic origin. Polymorphism of the CYP3A5 enzyme is much more common and occurs in approximately 10-20 percent of Caucasians, 33 percent of Japanese and 55 percent of African-Americans.[151] The majority of the genetic variation in CYP3A5 results in a poor-metabolizer variant.[152] The clinical significance of the CYP3A5 enzyme overall is rather spotty at best.[153] There are studies, however, that indicate those of African ancestry have a higher prevalence of rapid metabolizing CYP3A5 alleles which does hold clinical significance.[154][155][156] Recent studies have shown that the CYP3A5*3 variant can have a major impact on the metabolism of drugs such as cyclosporine, nifedipine, verapamil, and tacrolimus. CYP3A5 Normal Metabolizers constitute the minority in European populations. CYP3A4 Poor Metabolizers are rare, and absence of functional CYP3A5 is the norm in many populations. This is most notable for Caucasians with 80-85 percent of the population being homozygous for the variant CYP3A5*3 allele.[157] Genotyping of the CYP3A5 enzyme, however, should not replace therapeutic drug monitoring, as other factors (i.e. demographic factors, drug-drug interactions, genetic variation affecting a drug's pharmacodynamics) also influence a drug's dose requirements.

Testing separately for CYP 3A4/3A5 enzymes should only be done if there is clearly a unique situation that warrants it – such as a patient with a history of experiencing adverse effects with medications which are primarily metabolized by these enzymes. Most of the time, the genotyping of these enzymes should be ordered in conjunction with clinical evidence supporting genotyping for CYP2D6 polymorphisms with a clear secondary clinical impact of CYP3A4/3A5 polymorphisms.[158][159][160] As a rule the evidence supports ordering a CYP3A4/3A5 genotyping and phenotyping assay in patients of Japanese and African ancestry who have experienced a pattern of adverse drug reactions or have not responded to treatment.[161][162]

The tables below give information only related to CYP3A4 given the low clinical utility of CYP3A5 for psychiatry at this time. As you can see, the high-capacity / low affinity CYP3A4 enzyme is, by far, the enzyme most involved in the metabolization of medications. In the majority of cases, it acts as a secondary metabolizer. The clinical utility of this enzyme increases linearly with the number of medications and/or vitamin supplements a patient is taking. The sheer number of possible interactions with substrates of CYP3A4 emphasizes the importance of coordinating care with other providers and specialists.

Medications Metabolized by CYP3A4 (Substrates)
*medications of most importance to psychiatry are in blue

Alfentanil (Alfenta)	Erythromycin	Praziquantel (Biltricide)
Alfuzosin (Uroxatral)	Estazolam (ProSom)	Prednisolone
Almotriptan (Axert)	Estradiol	Prednisone
Alprazolam (Xanax)	Eszopiclone (Lunesta)	Progesterone
Amiodarone (Cordarone)	Ethosuximide (Zarontin)	Propanolol (Inderal)
Amlodipine (Norvasc)	Etoposide (Vepesid)	Propoxyphene (Darvon)
Aprepitant (Emend)	Exemestane (Aromasin)	Quazepam (Doral)
Aripiprazole	Felodipine (Plendil)	Quetiapine (Seroquel)
Astemizole	Fentanyl (Sublimaze)	Quinacrine
Atazanavir (Reyataz)	Finasteride (Proscar)	Quinidine
Atorvostatin (Lipitor)	Flurazepam (Dalmane)	Quinine
Bepridil (Vascor)	Fosamprenavir (Lexiva)	Ranolazine (Ranexa)
Bexarotene (Targretin)	Galantamine (Reminyl)	Repaglinide (Prandin)
Bosentan (Tracleer)	Gefinitib (Iressa)	Rifabutin (Rimactane)
Bromocryptine (Parlodel)	Granisetron (Kytril)	Risperidone (Risperdal)
Buprenorphine (Subutex)	Haldoperidol (Haldol)	Ritonavir (Norvir)
Buspirone (Buspar)	Holofantrine (Halfan)	Salmeterol (Serevent)
Carbamazepine (Tegretol)	Hydrocortisone	Saquinavir (Invirase)
Cevimeline (Evoxac)	Ifosfamide (Ifex)	Sibutramine (Meridia)
Chlorpheniramine	Imatinib (Gleevec)	Sildenafil (Viagra)
Cilostazol (Pletal)	Indinavir (Crixivan)	Simvastatin (Zocor)
Cisapride (Propulsid)	Irinotecan (Camptosar)	Sirolimus (Rapamune)
Clarithromycin (Biaxin)	Isradipine (DynaCirc)	Solifenacin (Vesicare)
Clonazepam (Klonopin)	Itraconazole (Sopranos)	Sorafenib (Nexavar)
Clopidogrel (Plavix)	Ixabepilone (Ixampra)	Sufentanil (Sufenta)
Cocaine	Ketoconazole (Nizoral)	Sunitinib (Sutent)
Colchicine	Lapatinib (Tykerb)	Tacrolimus (Prograf)
Cyclophosphamide (Cytoxan)	Levomethadyl (Orlaam)	Tadalafil (Cialis)
Cyclosporine (Neoral)	Lidocaine	Tamoxifen (Nolvadex)

Dapsone (Avlosulfon)	Loperamide (Imodium)	Tamsulosin (Flomax)
Darunavir (Prezista)	Loratadine (Claritin)	Telithromycin
Dasatinib (Sprycel)	Lovastatin (Mevacor)	Telithromycin
Delavirdine (Rescriptor)	Maraviroc (Selzentry)	Teniposide (Vumon)
Dextromethorphan	Methadone	Terfenadine
Dexamethasone (Decadron)	Methylprednisolone	Testosterone
Diazepam	Midazolam (Versed)	Tiagabine (Gabitril)
Dihydroergotamine	Modafinil (Provigil)	Tinidazole (Tindamax)
Diltiazem (Cardizem)	Nefazodone	Tipranavir (Aptivus)
Disopryamide (Norpace)	Nelfinavir	Tirazolam
Docetaxel (Taxotere)	Nevirapine (Viramune)	Topiramate (Topamax)
Domperidone	Nicardipine (Cardene)	Trazodone (Desyrel)
Donepezil (Aricept)	Nifedipine (Adalat)	Triazolam (Halcion)
Doxorubicin (Adriamycin)	Nimodipine (Nimotop)	Vardenafil (Levitra)
Droperidol	Nitrendipine (Baypress)	Verapamil (Calan)
Dutasteride (Avodart)	Odansetron (Zofran)	Vinblastine (Velbane)
Ebastine (Kestine)	Oxybutynin (Ditropan)	Vincristine (Oncovin)
Efavirenz (Sustiva)	Oxycodone (Percodan)	Ziprasidone (Geodon)
Elitryptan (Relpax)	Paclitaxel (Taxol)	Zolpidem (Ambien)
Eplerenone (Inspra)	Paricalcitol (Zemplar)	Zonisamide (Zonegram)
Ergotamine (Ergomar)	Pimozide (Orap)	Zopiclone (Imovane)
Erlotinib (Tarceva)	Pioglitazone	

Medications that Inhibit CYP3A4 (Inhibitors)

*medications of most importance to psychiatry are in blue

Amiodarone	Imatinib
Amprenavir	Indinavir
Aprepitant	Isoniazid
Atazanavir	Itraconazole
Chloramphenicol	Ketoconazole
Cimetidine	Laptinib
Ciprofoxacin	Miconazole
Clarithromycin	Nefazodone
Conivaptan	Nelfinavir
Cyclosporine	Norfloxacin
Darunavir	Posaconazole
Dasatinib	Ritonovir
Delavirdine	Quinupristin
Diltiazem	Saquinavir
Erythromycin	Tamoxofen
Fluconazole	Telithromycin
Fluoxetine (Prozac)	Troleandomycin
Fluvoxamine (Luvox)	Verapamil
Grapefruit Juice	Voriconazole

Medications that Induce CYP3A4 (Inducers)

*medications of most importance to psychiatry are in blue

Aminoglutethimide	Nevirapine
Barbiturates (Phenobarbital)	Oxcarbazepine (Trileptal)
Bexatrotene	Phenytoin (Dilantin)
Bosentran	Primidone
Carbamezepine (Tegretol)	Rifabutin
Dexamethasone	Rifampin
Efavirenz	Rifapentine
Fosphenytoin	St. John's Wort
Glucocorticoids	
Griseofulvin	
Modafinil	
Nafcillin	

The table below shows the allele frequency of CYP3A5*3.[163] [164] [165] Other or rarer variants are not included due to variance in frequencies and/or unknown clinical significance.

Allele	Enzyme Activity	Ethnic Background			
		Caucasian	Asian	Middle Eastern	African American
*3	Decreased	92%	74%	88%	32%

Our analysis on the same population of 14,615 patients for the CYP3A5 enzyme included variants of the *3 allele. A significantly large percentage of the subjects – 72.3 percent – were categorized as poor metabolizers.

The tested CYP3A5 phenotypic frequency of the mixed-race, U.S. based patients is shown below[166].

CYP3A5 Phenotype	Prevalence
Normal Metabolizer	7.2%
Intermediate Metabolizer	20.5%
Poor Metabolizers	72.3%

CLINICAL CASES IN PSYCHIATRIC PHARMACOGENETICS CASES FROM THE CLINIC AND HOSPITAL

Case 1: CYP2C19 Normal Metabolizer
CYP2D6 Ultra Rapid Metabolizer
CYP2C9 Intermediate metabolizer

Key Medications Involved: Buprenorphine, Bupropion Hydrochloride (Wellbutrin), Buproprion Hydrobromide (Aplenzin), Vilazidone (Viibryd)

This patient is a fifty-one year-old Latin-American female with a lifelong history of depression and co-morbid anxiety. She has been in recovery from opioid dependence for five years. She was labeled "treatment refractory and possibly treatment resistant" by her former attending psychiatrist in California. She has been prescribed, and failed to respond to, Celexa (CYP2C19 substrate), Prozac (primary CYP2D6 substrate; CYP2C19 inhibitor), Paxil (primary CYP2D6 substrate), Zoloft (CYP2C19 substrate), Cymbalta (primary CYP2D6 substrate), and more recently Lexapro (primary CYP2C19 substrate). Her records and her subjective report indicated she began to have signs of a response with Buproprion (CYP2D6 hepatic / CYP2B6 brain substrate) in the past. Her thyroid function tests, B12, RBC Folate, 25-OH Vitamin D and gonadal panel were all normal. Given that she had failed numerous antidepressant trials, Cytochrome P450 genotyping and phenotyping was ordered and the results returned as follows: CYP2C19 Normal Metabolizer, CYP2D6 Ultra Rapid Metabolizer, and CYP2C9 Intermediate Metabolizer. Upon a more detailed review of her records, it was confirmed she was prescribed Buproprion while she was also being treated for opioid dependence with Buprenorphine (Suboxone; CYP3A4 substrate and CYP2D6 inhibitor). At a dose of 300mg XL brand Wellbutrin she started feeling better. One month thereafter she completed her treatment for opiate dependence and Buprenorphine was tapered and discontinued. She soon complained of feeling depressed. Wellbutrin is increased to 450mg, with no significant improvement. It was decided to taper her off Wellbutrin. A trial of Viibryd

(Vilazodone; CYP3A4 substrate and minor inducer of CYP2C19) was started. At 40mg, she started showing a clinical response. Montgomery-Asberg Depression Rating Scores (MADRS) decreased from 41 to 34 and then to 30 within the first four weeks. After about three months of treatment on 40mg of Viibryd, there was no change in her reported symptoms or MADRS scores. Simultaneously, she received individual psychotherapy. Viibryd was augmented with low dose Liothyronine (T3; not metabolized by CYP450 system) which was titrated to 50mcg daily within five weeks. Her MADRS score decreased to 23 at six months. Per protocol, Liothyronine was tapered at eight weeks. Vibryd was continued at 40mg, and Aplenzin (Buproprion Hydrobromide) was started and titrated to 522mg. Her MADRS score decreased to 18 about four weeks after starting Aplenzin. They remained at 18 for about two more months and then reduced further to 12. It was then discovered her depression was much more severe during winter months. Starting in October, she began augmenting her psychotropic regimen with chronotherapy (UV-B broad spectrum light) every morning for 30 minutes. She stops using her light box in early April. Her average MADRS score eventually dropped to a 6 and she has been in remission now for fourteen months.

DISCUSSION: This patient is a CYP2D6 Ultra-Rapid Metabolizer. Buprenorphine is highly protein bound and is primarily metabolized by CYP3A4. It is also a potent inhibitor of CYP3A4 and a potent inhibitor of CYP2D6. Bupropion is metabolized by CYP2B6, in the brain and CYP2D6 in the liver. When this patient was taking Buprenorphine, it inhibited the metabolization of Buproprion and, thus, most likely allowed it to accumulate at levels that fostered a clinical response. Aplenzin – Buproprion Hydrobromide – undergoes the same CYP450 metabolization as Wellbutrin – Buproprion Hydrochloride. In essence, the presence of Buprenorphine allowed relatively normal CYP2D6 action with regard to its action on Bupropion. When Buprenorphine was discontinued, the CYP2D6 enzyme ultra-rapid action was then 'unmasked' and Bupropion levels dropped significantly. The initiation of Viibryd was a very good choice as it is metabolized via the CYP3A4 enzymatic pathway (and is a minor inducer of CYP2C19). The use of Liothyronine (Cytomel) is an old trick in psychiatry to 'boost' the action of a given antidepressent – in this case, Viibryd. Liothyronine completely bypasses the Cytochrome P450 system.

Case 2: CYP2C19 Normal Metabolizer
CYP2D6 Normal Metabolizer
CYP2C9 Poor Metabolizer

Key Medications Involved: Phenytoin, Valproate, Olanzapine

This patient is a thirty-seven year-old female with a diagnosis of unspecified Bipolar Disorder and Partial Complex Seizures. Her seizures has been well managed on Dilantin (Phenytoin; metabolized by CYP2C9 and CYP2C19) for a number of years with static average blood levels of 14 to 16 mcg/mL. She suffered her first overtly manic episode and was taken to the local emergency room. She was found to be volume depleted and in moderate acute renal failure and was admitted to the internal medicine service. Her serum Dilantin level on admission was 10 mcg/mL and it was discovered through a collateral source of information that she had not likely taken her medication in several days as she felt she had "cured herself" of seizures. Her last witnessed seizure was about 2 years prior. The attending internist re-started her out-patient dose of Dilantin and requested a psychiatric consult. The attending psychiatrist recognized overt symptoms of mania – patient was observed to displayed very rapid speech, ruminative thought processes, grandiosity and was repeatedly attempting to leave the hospital. She was started on Zyprexa (Olanzapine; metabolized by CYP1A2 and to a lesser extent by CYP2D6 and CYP3A4) for acute management of her mania. Lithium was considered for maintenance treatment, but was contraindicated due to her acute renal failure. She was started on Depakote ER (minimal substrate of CYP2C9 but strong inhibitor of the same) and, over about a week's time, the dose was titrated to 500mg twice daily. Her symptoms of mania resolved within 48 hours. On the sixth day of her hospitalization, the attending internist noticed the patient was rather confused and dysphasic. The on-call neuropsychiatrist was called. Upon examination, it was clear the patient was moderately confused, had slowed thinking, and rather stilted speech with word-finding deficits. Additionally, she was observe to have horizontal beating nystagmus and a mild tremor as well. Her reflexes were hyporeflexia throughout. She had mild gingival hyperplasia – a rather common phenomenon in patients on long term Dilantin treatment. The patient's pupils were a bit large but equal, round and reactive. There was no focal neurological signs.

Stat *free* Dilantin and *free* Valproate levels were ordered, as was a serum NH+3 (Ammonia). Available lab results were reviewed. The patient's renal function had normalized and her Albumin was low normal. Her PT/PTT were normal. Her liver enzymes were normal. Her CBC showed some eosinophilia and borderline megaloblastic anemia. Intravenous normal saline was increased from 75cc/hour to 150cc/hour. A Cytochrome P450 Genotyping and Phenotyping assay was ordered and the results followed: CYP2C19 Normal Metabolizer, CYP2D6 Normal Metabolizer and CYP2C9 Poor Metabolizer. Free Dilantin levels returned as toxic. Free Valproate levels returned as borderline toxic. The patient's NH3+ level returned elevated at 43, which was essentially clinically irrelevant. The patient's Dilantin was held for thirty-six hours and then resumed at 25% of her previous dose. Depakote was held for 24 hours and re-started at 250mg twice daily. In one week Depakote was increased to 500mg twice daily and Olanzapine was tapered. One week thereafter the patient's free and total Dilantin levels were therapeutic and her Depakote level returned as low-normal/therapeutic. There were no symptoms of mania, and her symptoms of Dilantin toxicity had completely resolved. This patient has been stable for the past ten months with no emergent symptoms of mania or depression. Her Dilantin and Depakote levels have been therapeutic.

DISCUSSION: This patient had classic signs and symptoms of Phenytoin toxicity. Eosinophilia and megaloblastic anemia can occur with long-term use of this medication. Eosinophilia tends to be more common with acute toxicity. Phenytoin is metabolized by the cytochrome P450 enzymes CYP2C9 and CYP2C19. Valproate (Depakote/Valproic Acid) is not only an inhibitor of CYP2C9 but is highly protein bound. The metabolization of Valproate is complicated with at least three pathways involved. The two primary routes are glucoronidation and beta oxidation in the mitochondria, with about 10 percent being metabolized by CYP2C9. Phenytoin is also highly protein bound. Both drugs probably were knocking each other off proteins and thus increasing free drug levels. The crucible event was likely the inhibition of CYP2C9 which significantly increased free Phenytoin levels into the toxic range, thereby producing classic physical signs and symptoms of Phenytoin toxicity. In addition, the patient's CYP2C9 poor metabolizer status caused a reduced clearance of Phenytoin and, thus, only added to toxic serum levels. Olanzapine is metabolized primarily by direct glucuronidation and CYP1A2 and to a lesser extent by CYP2D6 and CYP3A4.

Case 3: CYP2C9 Normal Metabolizer
CYP2D6 Normal metabolizer
CYP2C19 Rapid metabolizer

Key Medications Involved: Aripiprazole, Fluoxetine

This patient is a fifty two year-old Caucasian female with diagnosis of type II Bipolar Disorder with soft psychotic features limited to chronic intermittent generalized paranoia with no bizarre characteristics. She has had a history of only partially responding to psychotropic treatment in the past. From the patient's subjective report, a detailed review of records, and her current attending psychiatrist's discussion with two of her former treating psychiatrists, it was confirmed that she failed treatment with Valproic Acid, Carbamazepine, Clomipramine, Citalopram, and Buproprion. She did start to respond to Symbyax (Olanzapine-Fluoxetine combination) within approximately ten days after initiating treatment, however, the patient gained considerable weight and was persistently hyperglycemic, so this medication was discontinued. The patient then responded to a trial of Abilify (a primary CYP2D6 and secondary CYP3A4 substrate) 10mg qHS, and was in partial remission for approximately 4 months before her symptoms of depression re-emerged. Cytochrome CYP450 genotyping and phenotyping was ordered and the results were as follows: CYP2C9 Normal Metabolizer, CYP2D6 Normal metabolizer, and CYP2C19 Rapid Metabolizer. Abilify was increased to 15mg, however, her insurance company denied coverage for unknown reasons. The patient was then provided samples of 5mg to accompany the 10mg dose her insurance company covered. In approximately ten days, the patient's symptoms began to improve. After discussing some creative options with her, Fluoxetine (Prozac) was prescribed at 20mg q/day (predominantly metabolized by CYP2D6 and secondarily by CYP3A4; inhibitor of CYP2C19, CYP2C9, and CYP3A4). The 10mg dose of Abilify was continued, and the additional 5mg Abilify office sample was stopped. To reduce the risk of akathisia, the patient was instructed to take Fluoxetine daily, but to take Abilify on alternating days.[167] The patient was seen weekly and the dose of Fluoxetine was increased to 40mg. At 40mg of Fluoxetine plus 10mg of Abilify daily the patient's symptoms completely resolved. She has been in remission now for one year which is the longest period of remission for her to date.

DISCUSSION: The rationale behind prescribing Fluoxetine was simple. In additional to typical symptoms of depression, this patient's symptoms of depression included a predominance of modest psychomotor retardation, deficits in executive function (e.g. explicit memory, concentration, planning, interest, motivation), and mild word-finding deficits. The organicity of her symptoms indicated a predominant problem with her dopaminergic circuitry (see research by Yale Un. and Un. of Toronto, as well as Jan Faucett, MD at the Un. of New Mexico on the role of dopamine in depression subtypes). Fluoxetine was not prescribed for depression. It was prescribed as a metabolic inhibitor of the CYP2D6 pathway to subsequently increase active Aripiprazole and Dihydro-Aripiprazole levels. This pragmatic approach saved both time and money.[168] Fluoxetine is predominantly metabolized by CYP2D6 and to a lesser extent CYP3A4. About 10 percent of the drug is excreted unchanged in the urine. It is important to know that it is an inhibitor of CYP2C19, CYP2C9, and CYP3A4.

Case 4: CYP2C9 Normal Metabolizer
CYP2D6 Intermediate Metabolizer
CYP2C19 Rapid Metabolizer

Key Medications Involved: Duloxetine, Dexamphetamine (Adderall)

This patient is a seventeen year-old Caucasian female who had previously seen physicians at the Mayo Clinic in Scottsdale, Arizona and Baylor Medical Center in Houston, Texas. Her parents were both supportive, intelligent people who were very concerned about their daughter. She initially presented with almost two years of generalized weakness, lower extremity paresthesia, anesthesia and episodes of cataplexy (aka 'drop attacks'). Her 'drop attacks' came suddenly and without warning and, as a result, she had hit her head several times and had broken her collarbone on one occasion. Her weakness and frequency of cataplexy has progressed so much that she was in a wheelchair most of the time. In addition, she described having "seizures" which manifested as her eyes rolling back and her being unaware of her surroundings for, on average, one to four minutes. Her parents reported their daughter would appear rather dazed and somewhat confused thereafter. A previous 72-hour video-assisted EEG as well as a polysomnogram at Mayo Clinic the year before had been negative for both seizure activity and narcolepsy. Subsequent MRIs of her brain at both Mayo Clinic and Baylor Medical Center were also unremarkable. Two consulting neurologists from each respective institution had essentially reported her to be neurologically healthy. The psychiatrist's first order of action was to request that her parents videotape all incidents, to implement fall precautions at her home (to include placing her mattress on the floor). The patient was asked to keep a daily journal of her symptoms. Cytochrome P450 genotyping and phenotyping was ordered, and the results returned as CYP2C9 Normal Metabolizer, CYP2D6 Intermediate Metabolizer, and CYP2C19 Rapid Metabolizer. The suddenness of her cataplexy and the fact it had caused numerous falls and trauma in the past, and had markedly limited her life, was very concerning, so she was started on a course of Adderall XR 5mg (Dexamphetamine XR; substrate and inhibitor of CYP2D6) every morning and was asked to start using a four-legged ('quad') walker when she ambulated at home. Over approximately three months, her dose of Dexamphetamine XR was increased to 10mg and then to 15mg respectively. The frequency of her cataplexy improved dramatically after starting Dexamphetamine. A low-dose of Gabapentin –100mg TID – was started to help her paresthesia/anesthesia as well as to help her anxiety (bypasses CYP450 metabolization and excreted renally).

Approximately six months after starting Dexamphetamine, Cymbalta (predominantly metabolized by CYP2D6 and, to a minor extent, CYP1A2; inhibitor of CYP2D6) was initiated at 20mg daily to help with symptoms of reactive depression – which were quite understandable as she was essentially sequestered from her friends and high school and, in essence, a normal teenage experience. Within one week of starting Cymbalta, the patient complained of headache and "feeling shaky". At her next follow-up visit, her normally low baseline blood pressure was observed to be increased from 106/60 to 128/74. Dexamphetamine XR was reduced from 15mg to 5mg and her headaches and shakiness resolved within thirty-six hours and her blood pressure returned to her normal baseline. She was allowed an as-needed dose of 5mg immediate-release Dexamphetamine tablets in the late afternoon. She showed further improvement over the next three months, however, she continued to have "seizures" with post-event confusion. A repeat 72-hour video-assisted EEG was, again, negative for seizure activity with no electrophysiological evidence of narcolepsy.

Throughout this time, her parents and psychiatrist viewed many hours of video which verified there was a predominance of atypical symptoms – nonetheless with some typical symptoms - of a seizure disorder. Her cataplexy had yet to fully resolve as she continued to have a few episodes weekly. Prior to this, she did not seem keen on engaging in intensive psychotherapy, however, by continual gentle coaxing she finally agreed. It was revealed that, at age 14, she had been raped. She had never told anyone. She had not even informed her parents, with whom she told everything to. At this point, it was suspected that there were two likely processes occurring simultaneously: one was a supra-tentorial conversion disorder, the other was a real organic medical problem. Over the next several visits, this patient completed orthostatic vital measurements and it was discovered she was chronically, and quite markedly, orthostatic. This information was conveyed to her pediatrician, who started her on a course of Midodrine (CYP2D6 inhibitor) while her psychiatrist slowly tapered her off Vyvanse (Lisdexamphetamine). Her daily water intake had been verified to be quite substantial. At the request of her psychiatrist, she began seeing a very skilled hypnotherapist. Within three months her 'seizures' were occurring infrequently and her cataplexy was nearly gone. Within eight months her seizures were only occurring on the average of once monthly and her cataplexy completely resolved.

DISCUSSION: This young lady is about as complex a psychiatric patient as you get. In such cases, details are critically important. A person's "intermediate metabolizer' status should not be overlooked. This patient was exhibiting quit clear symptoms of a drug-drug interaction between Adderall XR (Dexamphetamine) and Cymbalta (Duloxetine). Both Dexamphetamine and Duloxetine are substrates of the CYP2D6 enzyme. To a much lesser extent, Duloxetine is also a secondary substrate of CYP1A2. Even at an intermediate metabolizer status, this patient's serum dexamphetamine level increased. Just as important is the fact that Duloxetine is a moderate inhibitor of the CYP2D6 enzyme. When Dexamphetamine XR was reduced back to 5mg every morning, her shakiness and hypertension resolved. Midrodine is a comparably mild non-competitive inhibitor of CYP2D6. It is not, however, metabolized by the CYP450 system. Instead, it is thought to undergo deglycination to desglymidodrine in numerous tissues.

Case 5: CYP2C19 Poor Metabolizer
CYP2C9 Normal Metabolizer
CYP2D6 Intermediate Metabolizer

Key Medications Involved: Amitriptyline, Nortriptyline, Fluoxetine, Propanolol, Diazepam

This patient is a forty two year-old Caucasian female with a diagnosis of recurrent major depression with comorbid panic disorder. She is also a type II diabetic with mild lower extremity neuropathy. Upon initial consultation, her psychotropic medications included Amitripyline 150mg at bedtime (minor portions metabolized by CYP2C19, secondarily, CYP2D6), Fluoxetine 80mg every morning (CYP2D6 substrate and strong inhibitor), Gabapentin 300mg four times daily (not metabolized by CYP450 system), and Diazepam 5mg twice daily (primary substrate of CYP2C19). Her diabetic medications included Metformin 1000mg twice daily. Her blood pressure was slightly elevated at 138/71 with mild tachycardia at 104 beats per minute. Her neurological exam was unremarkable. Her precordial exam was notable for tachycardia, but with no appreciable murmurs, clicks or rubs. She complained of intermittent chest pain she attributed to her panic attacks, but did note that her chest pain seemed to persist for a while, at times, after the remainder of her panic symptoms subsided. She denied any concomitant radiation to her anterior neck, jaw, arm or hand. Her principal complaint during this initial visit was anxiety, fragmented and non-restful sleep and intermittent panic attacks. A CYP450 genotyping and phenotyping assay was ordered for CYP2D6/2C19/2C9 as well as labs for serum B12, Folic Acid, 25-OH Vitamin D and Thyroid Function Studies (TSH, Free T3 and Free T4). Her B12 returned normal, but her folic acid returned a bit low at 5 ng/ml. Her active Vitamin D was normal as were her Thyroid Function Studies. Pharmacogenetic testing results returned as CYP2C19 Poor Metabolizer, CYP2C9 Normal Metabolizer, and CYP2D6 Intermediate Metabolizer. At this visit serum Amitriptyline and Nortriptyline levels were ordered as well as an EKG. While awaiting the results, Amitriptyline was reduced from 125mg to 75mg at bedtime and Fluoxetine was reduced from 80mg to 40mg daily (60mg a/day x week 1 then 40mg q/day thereafter). Her

Amitriptyline level returned at 330 ng/mL – 30 units into the toxic range. Her Nortryptiline (predominantly metabolized by CYP2D6) level returned at 190 ng/ml, which is not quite toxic, but about 10 to 20 units above the maximal recommended therapeutic range for Nortryptiline. Her EKG showed a mildly widened QRS complex and an increased QTc interval. Her Amitryptiline was held for 72 hours and then re-started at 50mg at bedtime. Propanolol LA 80mg (primary substrate of CYP2D6) was started every morning and a low dose of Clonazepam was started at 0.5mg twice daily (primary substrate of CYP3A4). Within two weeks, this patient's anxiety was markedly improved. A repeat serum Amitryptline level returned as therapeutic at 200 ng/ml. A repeat EKG was normal and her vitals were normal. To be cautious, a cardiology consult was requested to evaluate her chest pain that persisted after her panic attack.

DISCUSSION: This patient's anxiety and panic symptoms are likely worsened from toxic levels of Amitryptiline. Approximately 90 percent of Amitryptiline is protein bound. A large portion of it (50 percent or more) is demethylated in the liver to its primary metabolite Nortryptiline. The remainder is excreted in the urine as glucuronide or sulfate conjugate of metabolites, with little unchanged drug appearing in the urine. Small amounts are excreted in feces via biliary elimination. It is thought that perhaps 25 percent is metabolized by CYP2C19. Nortryptiline, however, is primarily metabolized by CYP2D6. As Fluoxetine is a major inhibitor of CYP2D6, this enzyme could not be adequately engaged in this case to help metabolize Amitryptiline's intermediate metabolite Nortryptiline. In addition, CYP2C19 is secondarily involved in the metabolization of Amitryptiline. Lowering the dose of Amitryptiline from 150mg to 50mg was, thus, clearly a prudent decision. The addition of Propanolol was, in hindsight, probably unnecessary, however, given it is metabolized by the CYP2D6 enzyme – as are beta-blockers – appeared to have a positive effect on her panic attacks. It could also useful in helping her taper off Diazepam as this medication is primarily metabolized by CYP2C19 and, even at 5mg twice daily, has a significant risk of instigating adverse effects. Having chest pain that persists after her panic symptoms have resolved is unusual and usually indicative of angina, ischemia or a tachyarrhythmia such as this patient was experiencing, thus it was very appropriate to request a cardiology consult. Clonazepam is primarily metabolized by CYP3A4.

Case 6: CYP2C9 Normal Metabolizer
CYP2C19 Ultra Rapid Metabolizer
CYP2D6 Intermediate Metabolizer

Key Medications Involved: Venlafaxine, Buproprion, Diazepam, Topiramate

This patient is a forty-seven year-old Hispanic female with a history of Generalized Anxiety Disorder and Tonic-Clonic Seizures. She also suffers from Gastro-Esophageal Reflux Disease (GERD) and comorbid chronic back pain residual to two lumbar laminectomies in the past. Her psychotropic medications at her initial consult include Diazepam 10mg four times daily (primary substrate of CYP2C19), Topamax (Topiramate; a minor amount is metabolized by CYP3A4) 200mg twice daily (not significantly metabolized by the CYP450 system), Effexor XR (Venlafaxine ER; principal substrate of CYP2D6) 150mg twice daily and Buproprion SR 200mg every morning (principal substrate of CYP2D6 and (CYP2B6 in the brain). In addition, she was taking Protonix 40mg daily (principal substrate of CYP2C19). Formal mental status testing revealed an anxious female who looked older than her stated age. She was fidgety and her span of attention was a bit scattered. Her thought processes were ruminative. She had modest deficits in her explicit memory. She endorsed being "anxious all the time...like I'm shaky anxious and can't sit still." She also complained of nausea. Her blood pressure was measured manually at176/86, and her pulse was 108. She confirmed she smokes approximately ½ pack per day, but stated her blood pressure "is usually in the 140s". She reported that, at times, she has shortness of breath. She endorsed significant trouble going to sleep. She had stopped consuming coffee lately "because it just made me more anxious and nauseated". She complained of short term memory loss which had progressed over the previous year. Her neurological examination was normal. Her precordial examination revealed two or three skipped beats in one minute but no murmurs, clicks or rubs. Cytochrome P450 genotyping and phenotyping was ordered as a drug-gene interaction was suspected given the fact she is on three medications that are either substrates or inhibitors of the CYP2D6 enzyme. Additionally, EKG and Thyroid Function Studies were ordered. Pharmacogenetic testing results were remarkable for a CYP2C9 Normal Metabolizer, a CYP2C19 Ultra-Rapid Metabolizer and a CYP2D6 Intermediate Metabolizer. Her Thyroid Function studies returned as normal. Her EKG showed sinus tachycardia and a slight right axis deviation. Given the patient was on a rather high dose of Diazepam (10mg four times daily) quantitative blood levels were drawn which returned in the low therapeutic - non-toxic - range.

Venlafaxine ER and Buproprion SR were reduced to 150mg and 200mg every morning respectively as they both increase noradrenaline activity and, thus, increase the risk of - or even be the cause of - tachycardia. An initial titration of Keppra (Levetiracitam; does not undergo CYP450 metabolization) was started and Topamax (Topiramate) was slowly tapered. Leveteracitam seemed an optimal choice as it is not metabolized by CYP450 enzymes and rarely causes cognitive or memory impairment. Leveteracitam was titrated to 1000mg twice daily over a 3 week period. A repeat EKG showed normal sinus rhythm, slight right axis deviation, but no other irregularities. The patient's pulse normalized but her blood pressure, however, remained elevated at 151/83. She followed up with her cardiologist who began treatment for this. Additionally, he discontinued Protonix and started her on Ranitidine which afforded her resolution of her nausea. Within the ensuing months, her anxiety showed moderate improvement, however, she continued to have intermittent panic attacks and sleep problems. Psychotherapy was initiated and a trial of Viibryd (substrate of CYP3A4 and minor inducer of CYP2C19) was started. She was tapered off Diazepam by utilizing a combination of Clonazepam (primary substrate of CYP3A4) and Buspar (primary substrate of CYP3A4). The patient's panic attacks and anxiety, to date, are greatly improved and she is progressing well in psychotherapy.

DISCUSSION: This case likely represents an exacerbation of anxiety with tachycardia and somatic symptoms suggestive of a drug-gene-drug interaction in the CYP2D6 pathway between Venlafaxine and Bupropion. Additionally, given that Protonix is a principal substrate of CYP2C19, and the fact the patient is an Ultra-Rapid CYP2C19 metabolizer, it was not effective in controlling this patient's acid reflux, therefore causing her nausea, and contributing to her chest pain and anxiety. Changing to medication that is not metabolized by the CYP450 system – Ranitidine –

was a wise decision. Venlafaxine is principally metabolized by the CYP2D6 enzyme. Buproprion is principally metabolized by BYP2B6, however, this enzyme so much resembles the molecular shape of the CYP2D6 enzyme that they are nearly interchangeable. Most importantly for this case, Buproprion is a strong inhibitor of CYP2D6. As a result of this inhibition, serum Venlafaxine levels likely increased by 30% or more, causing the patient to become hypertensive and have chest pains outside her characteristic panic symptoms. Less-than 20 percent of Topiramate is metabolized by CYP3A4. About 70 percent of it is eliminated unchanged in the urine. Diazepam at 10mg four times daily is generally considered a very high dose. It is not surprising that, despite her high dose of Diazepam, quantitative levels returned in the low therapeutic range given her CYP2C19 ultra-rapid metabolizer status. Her short term memory loss was likely due to her protracted anxiety. Viibryd is principally metabolized via the CYP3A4 enzyme, and is a minor inducer of CYP2C19. Clonazepam and Buspirone (Buspar) are primarily metabolized by CYP3A4.

Case 7: CYP2C9 Normal Metabolizer
CYP2C19 Normal Metabolizer
CYP2D6 Poor Metabolizer

Key Medications Involved: Sertraline, Desvanlafaxine (Pristiq), Buproprion, Tramadol

This patient is a sixty five year-old female who suffers from Dysthymic Disorder and Chronic Fatigue Syndrome, thought to be from a previous Epstein-Barre viral infection. She presented with worsening depression, low interest, low motivation, reduced appetite with a reported ten-pound weight loss over about 5 weeks. She is rather physically trim with a BMI of 23.7. Her blood pressure at her initial visit was 124/70 with a pulse of 77. Her neurological exam was normal. She is a non-smoker. She had been started on Lamictal (not metabolized by CYP450 enzymes) by her primary care physician two years ago as "she did not care to take an antidepressant". About four months ago, she agreed to start Sertraline at 50mg daily (principally metabolized by CYP2C19). Her mental status examination was remarkable for a depressed mood and a rather blunted affect. She was pensive and her speed of cognitive processing was a bit sluggish. Her Montgomery-Asberg Depression Rating Scale (MADRS) was 36, which is consistent with moderate to severe symptoms of depression. A review of her overall medication history revealed some spotty intolerance to a few medications – rash with Amoxicillin and "anxiety and shakiness" with Tramadol. The following labs were ordered: Serum B12, Folic Acid and 25-OH Vitamin D, TSH, Free T3, Free T4 and a CBC with Differential. Her family history revealed her sister also suffered from depression and responded well to Effexor (Venlafaxine; principally metabolized by CYP2D6). Sertraline was tapered and an initial trial of Effexor was initiated at 37.5mg daily. In two weeks the dose was increased to 75mg. At a follow-up visit one month later the patient reported she felt less depressed, and her MADRS score was measured as 30. Her initial labs returned as normal/unremarkable. She, however, reported feeling more anxious and stated she felt "shaky sometimes". She also started having headaches over the past week. A CYP450 genotyping and phenotyping assay was ordered for the CYP2D6/2C19/2C9 pathways.

Her results yielded the following pharmacogenetic profile: CYP2C9 Normal Metabolizer, CYP2C19 Normal Metabolizer, and CYP2D6 Poor Metabolizer.

In the ensuing three months, the patient reported feeling overall better than she had initially; however her MADRS scores fluctuated between 28 and 30, and showed no further improvement. After discussing options with the patient, she was transitioned to Pristiq (Desvenlafaxine; not a substrate of the CYP450 system and is renally excreted), and titrated to its maximal dose. Within approximately two months after her transition to Pristiq, her MADRS score reduced to 24. After discussing options for additional treatment with the patient, she agreed to start cognitive behavioral therapy. Additionally, a low dose of Bupropion SR (primary substrate of CYP2D6 in the liver and 2B6 in the brain) was started but ordered to be given every other day. In the two months that followed, the patient reported significant improvement in her symptoms, and her MADRS scores further reduced to 18 and finally 12.

DISCUSSION: The patient's history of experiencing adverse medication reaction to Tramadol is understandable as it is metabolized predominantly by CYP2D6 and, secondarily, CYP3A4. It should be noted that approximately 30 percent of the dose of Tramadol is excreted in the urine unchanged. Sertraline is principally metabolized by CYP2C19. Venlafaxine is a principal metabolite of CYP2D6. Changing to Pristiq (Desvanlafaxine) was a good tactical decision as it is the active metabolite of Effexor (Venlafaxine) and completely bypasses first-pass metabolism (CYP450) metabolism. Bupropion is principally metabolized by CYP2B6 enzyme, however, given this enzyme is nearly identical to CYP2D6, there is often extensive crossover. Dosing Buprorion every other day was a good strategy as Bupropion has a mean half-life of 14 hours, which would certainly be extended in poor metabolizers of CYP2D6. Lamotrigine (Lamictal) undergoes hepatic undergoes glucoronidation in the liver.

Case 8: CYP2C9 Normal Metabolizer
CYP2C19 Normal Metabolizer
CYP2D6 Rapid Metabolizer

Key Medications Involved: Duloxetine, Hydrocodone

This patient is a twenty-nine year-old Hispanic male who suffers from chronic anxiety and chronic pain from an old multi-level disc herniation from an oilfield injury he suffered five years earlier at age twenty-four. He was referred to psychiatry by his primary care physician to help manage chronic anxiety. At his initial evaluation, he complained of being anxious "all the time." He reported he remembered being somewhat of a "worrier as a child" but added he became "more anxious and tense" after his injury. He reported he has great difficulty remaining seated for long periods of time, endorsed "feeling fidgety all the time" and "worries about the small things." He stated his mind "has a hard time stopping" which he feels keeps him awake at night. He denied racing thoughts or symptoms that would suggest episodes of hypomania or mania. He reportedly has tried numerous SSRIs to include Paroxetine and Fluoxetine (both principally metabolized by CYP2D6). He stated "These didn't touch me". He stated he did feel some improvement with Diazepam and Lorazepam (not metabolized by the CYP450 system), however, his pain management physician tapered him off Lorazepam when he was started on opiate pain medicationsa few years ago. His current medications include Hydrocodone 5mg q 6 hours (primarily a substrate of CYP2D6 and, to a minor extent, a substrate of CYP3A4), Cyclobenzaprine 10mg q 6 hours (substrate of CYP1A2), Acetaminophen 1000mg at bedtime as-needed (very minor substrate of CYP2E1, CYP1A2 and CYP3A4). After the psychiatrist discussed options for treatment, the patient agreed to start Cymbalta 60mg daily (principal substrate of CYP2D6) with the option of titrating this medication to 60mg twice daily if necessary - which is considered the optimal pain modulation dose for this medication. The next week the patient calls and informs his psychiatrist he believes the medication (Cymbalta) is causing him to be "loopy and drunk". He is advised to hold the medication and come into the office. He arrives the next morning and the psychiatrist asks him if there had been any new changes to his medications. The patient reported his pain management doctor recently increased Hydrocodone from 5mg three times daily to 10mg three times daily with an additional 5mg daily as-needed dose for break-through pain. A brief neurological examination reveals the patient's pupils are rather small, but reactive, and his reflexes are a bit slow. The mental status exam reveals his cognitive processing speed to be modestly sluggish with a mild latency in his responses. During the review of systems the patient reported he has been rather constipated over the past few weeks. The psychiatrist feels it is warranted to order pharmacogenetic testing for CYP2D6, CYP2C19 and CYP2C9. The patient is advised to consume plenty of water and is re-started on Cymbalta 30mg daily and rescheduled to return in one week. Finally, the patient is strongly advised not to drive a car or operate dangerous machinery. In three days, the psychiatrist calls him on the telephone to see how he is doing and he reports he still feels "woozy and loopy". He returns for his scheduled visit five days later to review the pharmacogenetic testing results, which are as follows: the patient is a CYP2D6 Rapid Metabolizer, and a Normal Metabolizer in the CYP2C19 and CYP2C9 pathways. The psychiatrist calls the pain management physician and discusses the results. It is then decided to be prudent to reduce Hydrocodone to 5mg three times daily and discontinue Cyclobenzaprine. The pain management physician agrees with the psychiatrist's recommendation to increase Cymbalta to 60mg daily for the next two weeks then to 60mg twice daily thereafter. The patient is scheduled to follow-up with his psychiatrist in two weeks and with his pain management doctor in one week. In two weeks the patient returns and reports his symptoms are resolved. The examination that day shows his sensorium to be completely clear, his cognitive processing speed and reflexes to be normal, and his pupils to be of normal and equivocal size.

DISCUSSION: This patient's symptoms invariably arose from a drug-gene interaction, with consideration of a mild superimposed drug-drug interaction. He is a CYP2D6 Rapid Metabolizer. Hydrocodone is converted to Hydromorphone via the CYP2D6 enzyme. Hydromorphone is eight times more potent than Morphine. In Rapid Metabolizers, Hydrocodone undergoes this metabolic conversion at a very rapid rate and accumulates in body quickly, and was likely the source of this patient's symptoms. It is possible that Cymbalta, which also is predominantly metabolized by the CYP2D6 enzyme, acted as a competitive substrate to some extent, however, given the patient's symptoms and findings on neurological and mental status examinations, this effect was likely only very mild and not clinically relevant. Cyclobenzaprine is metabolized by P-Glycoprotein and CYP1A2. Discontinuing this medication was not a bad idea, given it only muddies the clinical picture and increases the risks associated with polypharmacy. As it is not a substrate or inhibitor, another prudent choice could be to simply lower the dose. Acetaminophen primarily is metabolized by hepatic conjugation, with an estimation of less-than 25 percent being metabolized by the CYP2E1, CYP1A2 and CYP3A4 enzymes. The CYP450 system is not thought to have any clinical utility with this medication.

Case 9: CYP2C9 Normal Metabolizer
CYP2C19 Normal Metabolizer
CYP2D6 Poor Metabolizer

Key Medications Involved: Sertraline, Escitalopram, Hydrocodone

This patient is a forty six year-old African-American female who suffers from Social Anxiety and chronic pain from complex regional trauma to her right lower extremity due to a motor vehicle accident whereby her leg was compressed for several hours. She was referred to psychiatry by her primary care physician to help manage her anxiety. The patient's pain management consultant also requested the psychiatrist to look at her current psychotropic medications and make any recommendations as to how they might be modified to help improve this patient's pain control. In the pain management physician's consult request, he states that this patient has been very compliant with her care. About two weeks prior to her initial visit with the psychiatrist, the patient's pain management physician started her on Sertraline (principal substrate of CYP2C19 but moderate inhibitor of CYP2D6). This SSRI was selected as the patient reported she suffered from some significant nausea with Cymbalta in the past, and had - in her early 20s - responded well to a year-long trial of Sertraline her family physician prescribed for her at that time. During her initial visit with the psychiatrist, the patient reported she has been prescribed Percocet 10/325mg every 6 to 8 hours for break through pain for the past year. In addition, she reported she has been on a Fentanyl transdermal patch for the past three years and is now on two 75mg patches every 72 hours. She reported her pain management physician changed her from Percocet to Hydrocodone (primary substrate of CYP2D6) 10mg every 6 to 8 hours about three months ago and explained to her that he felt the new evidence regarding the adverse effects of long-term Acetaminophen use was compelling enough to only use this medications for short term use. She reported over the past two weeks her pain has become worse. The only change to her medications in the past two weeks was the initiation of Sertraline (principal substrate of CYP2C19), whose dose had been increased to 100mg five days ago. The patient denied suffering any trauma during this period, and denied increased physical exertion. She denied using over-the-counter medications. Her psychiatrist recommended that Sertraline be tapered and the patient initiate a trial of Escitalopram (which is a principal substrate of CYP2C19). Sertraline was reduced to 50mg daily for one week then stopped. Escitalopram was initiated at 5mg daily and increased to 10mg daily during one week later. The patient then followed-up with her pain management physician, and completed a Phenotyping and Genotyping assay for the CYP2D6, CYP2C9 and CYP2C19 enzymes. After her results revealed the patient to be a CYP2D6 Poor Metabolizer, her pain pain management physician discontinued Hydrocodone and started her on Opana (Oxymorphone; not metabolized by the CYP450 system). Within days she reported improved pain control, reduced anxiety and a modest improvement sleep.

DISCUSSION: Sertraline is primarily metabolized by the CYP2C19 enzyme. Hydrocodone is predominantly metabolized into Hydromorphone via the CYPD6 enzyme. Hydromorphone is approximately 8 times the potency of Morphine and has much more analgesia than Hydrocodone. Given that this patient is a CYP2D6 poor metabolizer – at about a 50 percent, or more, slower rate than a normal metabolizer – the conversion of Hydrocodone to the more powerful Hydromorphone is substantially reduced. This is the likely reason this patient is reporting reduced analgesia. When the patient was switched to Hydromorphone, her pain resolved in short order. Hydromorphone does not undergo CYP450 metabolization. Instead, it undergoes hepatic reduction and conjugation with glucuronic acid to form both active and inactive products. In this particular case, the psychiatrist took a good course of action by recommending a medication – Escitalopram – that bypasses the CYP2D6 enzyme and does not inhibit this enzyme in any significant way.

Case 10: CYP1A2 Normal Metabolizer
CYP2D6 Normal Metabolizer
CYP3A4 Normal Metabolizer

Key Medications Involved: Olanzapine, Sertraline, Benadryl, Benztropine Carbamazepine is mentioned in the discussion

This patient is a thirty-eight year old Caucasian female with paranoid-type Schizophrenia. She has been stable on Olanzapine 20mg daily (metabolized by CYP1A2 and to a lesser extent by CYP2D6 and CYP3A4) for the past ten years and has not required hospitalization because of excellent out-patient management to include Assertive Community Treatment (ACT) team visits to her group home and regular follow ups with the Schizophrenia clinic at the local university. Additionally, she had never developed any extrapyramidal symptoms or dystonia on this dose. Her older sister reportedly had been a stabilizing force throughout her life, and her sudden and tragic death in a car accident instigated severe symptoms of depression in our patient. After making statements about harming herself, she was subsequently taken to the emergency room and admitted to the university psychiatry ward. It was reported in her admission records she smoked an average of one pack of cigarettes per day. Two days after admission, the patient started to complain of neck and back discomfort and stiffness. On day three she was observed to have abnormal oro-buccal movements. She was given a 50mg one time dose of oral Benadryl (substrate of CYP2D6 and potent inhibitor of the same) and her Olanzapine was reduce to 10mg qHS. She was also started on Benztropine 1mg qHS (is not believed to undergo CYP450 metabolization). Her symptoms substantially improved within two hours after receiving Benadryl and were observed to have resolved the next morning. She received bereavement counseling and started on Sertraline 50mg daily (primary substrate of CYP2C19). Her symptoms of depression were significantly within one week. She was discharged with a treatment plan that included weekly psychotherapy, Olanzapine 12.5mg qHS, Benztropine 1mg qHS, and Sertraline 50mg q/day. Throughout her hospitalization she was on a daily Nicotine patch which was discontinued on discharge as the patient reportedly had no interest in pursuing smoking cessation. At her two week follow-up visit, she reported some auditory chatter with staff observing her to be internal preoccupied at times. She verified she had returned to smoking an average of one pack of cigarettes daily. Her Olanzapine was increased back to 20mg daily. At her follow-up visit one month thereafter, her auditory chatter was noted to be resolved and she had returned to her pre-hospitalization baseline, albeit with some residual symptoms of depression. Her therapist noted she was making steady progress in her weekly psychotherapy sessions.

DISCUSSION: Olanzapine undergoes hepatic glucuronidation but is then predominantly metabolized by the CYP1A2 enzyme forming the intermediate metabolite *N*-desmethylolanzapine.[169] This patient, like many patients who suffer from Schizophrenia, smokes extensively – approximately one pack per day. There is growing evidence that Nicotine improves processing of auditory stimuli (sensory gating) in patients with schizophrenia and may lessen negative symptoms by increasing dopamine in the nucleus accumbens and the prefrontal and frontal cortex, which also has an anxiolytic effect by reducing the distractibility of internal stimuli.[170] Important to this case, the preservatives and byproducts in cigarettes - other than Nicotine itself - induce the CYP1A2 enzyme, therefore increasing the metabolization of Olanzapine, and effectively lowering it's serum level.[171] Even in normal metabolizers, this can be, and often is, clinically significant.[172] Within two days of admission, this patient developed symptoms of dystonia and oro-buccal dyskinesia as she was now no longer allowed to smoke. The administration of Benadryl helped improve her symptoms acutely, and the reduction of her dose of Olanzapine to essentially half resolved her symptoms relatively quickly (within three days). Benadryl is principally metabolized by CYP2D6 with secondary, but clinically insignificant, involvement of CYP1A2, CYP2C9, and CYP2C19. It is also a potent inhibitor of CYP2D6. In patients who are CYP2D6 poor metabolizers, Benadryl should be avoided. Benadryl should be used with great care in patients receiving other CYP2D6 substrates, especially those that also have CYP2D6 inhibitor properties due to the risk of toxicity. One could argue that the addition of Benztropine was unnecessary. Benztropine is not thought to undergo CYP450 metabolization and is primarily excreted in the urine.

It should be noted that researchers have observed other drug- drug-gene interactions with Olanzapine. Mäenpää and colleagues observed that concomitant treatment with the CYP1A2 inhibitor Fluvoxamine (Luvox) resulted in increased Olanzapine serum levels and decreased rates of clearance.[173] As an aside, it is good to also note that Carbamazepine is known to induce both CYP1A2 and CYP3A4 enzymes. Two teams of investigators found a decrease in serum Olanzapine levels when patients were treated concomitantly with this Carbamazepine.[174] [175]

Case 11: CYP2D6 Intermediate Metabolizer
CYP2C19 Normal Metabolizer
CYP2C9 Normal Metabolizer

Key Medications & Dietary Supplements Involved: Paroxetine, Escitalopram, Venlafaxine, Buproprion, Cyproheptadine (Periactin), Buspirone, Nefazodone, Mirtazepine, Amantadine, Yohimbine, Gingko Biloba, Bethanechol

This patient is a 31 y/o Caucasian female who is being treated for a single episode of major depression. She is physically very healthy, exercises religiously, and is a successful attorney. She has been in remission on brand Paxil 60mg for two years, however, during her most recent follow of visit, she reported becoming increasingly frustrated with her reduced libido (Paroxetine is principally metabolized by CYP2D6 and is also a potent inhibitor of the same). She reportedly has been dating her boyfriend now for one year and is concerned about their reduced frequency of physical intimacy reporting "I just can't get in the mood". She feels the culprit is Paxil. She is very hesitant to try another antidepressant medication or event lower the dose, noting it has been the most effective medication to date and she did not feel any symptomatic remission until a 60mg dose was prescribed. She had previously undertaken trials of Sertraline, Escitalopram (generic and brand Lexapro) and Venlafaxine. Her symptoms only partially improved with Sertraline and Escitalopram (both primary substrates of CYP2C19) and she experienced anxiety and tremors on Venlafaxine (a primary substrate of CYP2D6) as well as a moderate increase in her systolic blood pressure (from her average of 123/68 to 139/68). After discussing some options to help with her treatment (to include Buproprion, Periactin (Cyproheptadine), Nefazodone, Mirtazepine and Amantadine) she agreed to start a trial of daily Buproprion SR (a primary substrate of CYP2D6 and CYP2B6 in the brain and a potent inhibitor of CYP2D6). She is started on a dose of 150mg every morning. During a routine telephone follow-up conversation one week later, she reported feeling "jittery and wound up" and having difficulty sleeping. She also reported her face "feels hot all the time". On a positive note, she reported a mild increased interest in sexual interest but describes having anorgasmia. A review of her records revealed she completed a genotyping and phenotyping analysis of Cytochromes CYP2D6, CYP2C19 and CYP2C9 last year resulting in a CYP2D6 intermediate metabolizer phenotype as the only abnormal value. It is then recommended that she discontinue Buproprion and start low dose Periactin (Cyproheptadine) 2mg one hour prior to intercourse. She reports during her follow-up visit two week later her aforementioned symptoms had completely resolved and she believes Periactin is working well. She, however, then reports "feeling a little tired" approximately thirty minutes after taking the medication, but feels it is tolerable and wants to continue this course of treatment.

DISCUSSION: Paroxetine is the most likely culprit of this patient's reduced libido. Buproprion was not a bad choice to address this, however, both Paroxetine and Buproprion are metabolized principally by the Cytochrome CYP2D6 enzyme. Given she is an intermediate metabolizer in the CYP2D6 pathway, and given Paroxetine is both a substrate, and a potent inhibitor, of CYP2D6, both Paroxetine and Buproprion clearance are reduced. And to make things even more complicated, Buproprion is also a potent inhibitor of CYP2D6.[176] Thus, both Paroxetine and Bupropion serum levels are increased in this patient due to her intermediate metabolizer CYP2D6 phenotype, with Paroxetine and Buproprion levels being further increased because of both Buproprion's and Paroxetine's inhibition of the CYP2D6 enzyme. Although one could consider starting a trial of Buproprion at 75mg daily, a better course of action is to avoid this medication combination altogether. The same essential interaction would also occur with Fluoxetine and Buproprion. Even in CYP2D6 normal metabolizers, the combination of Buproprion and Paroxetine or Fluoxetine should be used very cautiously. Other treatment considerations of SSRI-induced sexual disinterest and anorgasmia include Periactin (Cyproheptadine), Buspirone, Nefazodone, Mirtazepine, Amantadine, Yohimbine (which is both an over-the-counter supplement and a prescribed medication), Gingko Biloba and Bethanacol. The rationale and mechanism of each of these medications thought to improve poor libido and anorgasmia related to SSRIs is explained below.[177]

Cyproheptadine is an antihistamine with anti-serotonergic properties that has been reported for many years reverse antidepressant-induced sexual dysfunction. About half is metabolized primarily by CYP3A4, and the remaining 40 to 50 percent is excreted unchanged in the urine. Effective doses range from 2mg to 16mg. Anorgasmia is the sexual side effect most often reported to be alleviated by cyproheptadine. Cyproheptadine is effective when taken either on an as-needed basis (typically, 1 to 2 hours before intercourse) or on a regular basis. The most common side effect reported by patients is excessive sedation that is dose-related. In addition, the reversal of the therapeutic effect of the antidepressant can also occur and is also dose-related. This occurs generally in doses of 4mg and above. Another side effect commonly reported is increased appetite. This medication should be used cautiously in patients with eating disorders. [178] [179] [180] [181]

Buspirone is a Serotonin-1A partial agonist. It is primarily metabolized by CYP3A4. Most patients prescribed Buspirone for SSRI-induced sexual dysfunction take it daily. The dosage is the same as that used to treat anxiety – 15mg to 60mg total daily dose. The mechanism of action of Buspirone thought to treat SSRI-induced sexual dysfunction is the stimulation of presynaptic autoreceptors or its alpha-2 antagonism instigating the reduction of serotonergic tone by this medication's primary metabolite 1-pyrimidinylpiperazine. [182]

Nefazodone is an old antidepressant with strong post-synaptic serotonergic antagonizing properties. It is also primarily metabolized by CYP3A4. It is un-related to SSRIs or SNRIs and most chemically related to Trazodone. It is considered a serotonin modulator. It is only available in its generic form as the brand name of this medication, Serzone, was discontinued more than twenty-five years ago for reportedly causing fulminant liver failure. The generic Nefazodone has proven to be quite safe. Case reports (mostly with Sertraline) indicate that a dose of 100mg to 150mg taken as-needed one hour prior to sexual activity greatly improves SSRI-induced anorgasmia. [183]

Mirtazepine is a tetracyclic antidepressant. It is highly protein bound at approximately 85%. It is metabolized primarily by CYP2D6 and, to a lesser extent, CYP3A4. Inhibitors of these isoenzymes, such as paroxetine and fluoxetine, cause modestly increased mirtazapine plasma concentrations (17 and 32%, respectively) but often without leading to clinically relevant consequences in patients that are CYP2D6 normal metabolizers.[184] In patients who are poor metabolizers, toxicity can occur and caution should be exercised. It is rather uncommonly used to treat SSRI-induced sexual side effects. When this medication is used in this capacity, it is generally prescribed at doses of 15mg at bedtime but sometimes is prescribed at doses of 7.5mg one hour prior to intercourse. Its most common side effect is sedation, which is well-known to most practitioners. It is thought to help reverse SSRI-induced sexual dysfunction by its presynaptic alpha-2 activity.[185]

Amantadine is a dopamine agonist. It is mostly excreted in the urine and does not interact with the CYP450 system. It is rather old medication used initially as an antiviral (mostly to treat Influenza) and as adjuvant treatment for Parkinson 's disease. Additionally, it is used in the addiction realm to help with methamphetamine cravings. A small number of case studies have shown it to help reverse SSRI-induced anorgasmia as dopamine is thought to be a key neurotransmitter that modulates both arousal and orgasm.[186] [187] [188]

Yohimbine/Yohimbe/Yohimbe Bark is an alkaloid agent extracted from the bark of Corynanthe yohimbi. It is metabolized primarily by CYP2D6 and, secondarily, by CYP3A4. It is also a moderate inhibitor of the CYP2D6 enzyme. Its effectiveness in treating SSRI-induced sexual dysfunction is thought to be its presynaptic alpha-2 adrenergic antagonism.[189] Commonly prescribed dosages range from 5.4mg daily to three times daily.[190] [191] [192] Side effects commonly reported include nausea, anxiety, sweating, facial flushing and urinary urgency. Yohimbe is available as an over-the-counter capsule or a tincture both are lower-potency than prescription.

Gingko Biloba is mostly known for its use as a memory enhancing supplement. It is significantly metabolized by CYP3A4 and is also a moderate inducer of this enzyme. Its ability to enhance memory has been proven by several studies over the past decade to be rather marginal. Its use as a rather safer agent to improve SSRI-induced sexual dysfunction has proven to be somewhat more effective. Doses start at 60mg twice daily and can be increased as tolerated to 120mg twice daily. Common side effects reported by patients include nausea, diarrhea and anxiety. Gingko has been proven to partially inhibit platelet binding. Thus, it should not be used in patients on anticoagulants or in patients with bleeding disorders. It should be used cautiously in the elderly and at lower doses. The mechanism thought to help improve SSRI-induced sexual dysfunction is by increasing blood flow to the pelvic region via local alpha reception modulation.[193] [194]

Bethanechol is a cholinergic agonist structurally related to acetylcholine. It does not cross the blood brain barrier and its mechanism in treating psychotropic related sexual side effects is at local level. It is a substrate of CYP3A4. It is most commonly used to treat post-surgical urinary retention. Its use in treating SSRI and even MAO-inhibitor induced sexual dysfunction is becoming more frequent. The mechanism by which Bechanechol helps in is by stimulating the parasympathetic nervous system which is a principal mechanism of orgasm and ejaculation. Typical doses are divided daily as 10mg or 20mg but case studies have reported efficacy and safety in doses as high as 120mg daily.[195] [196]

Case 12: CYP2D6 Normal Metabolizer
CYP2C19 Normal Metabolizer
CYP2C9 Normal Metabolizer

Key Medications Involved: Abilify Maintenna (Long-Acting Injectable), Latuda, Propanolol

This patient is a 43 year-old Norwegian-American male with a diagnosis of Schizoaffective Disorder. His psychiatrist recently started him on a monthly injection of 400mg Aripiprazole (Abilify) Maintenna (primary substrate of CYP2D6 and, secondarily, CYP3A4) about ten days ago. His depression had been in remission with Fluoxetine 60mg q/day for the past three years (primary substrate of CYP2D6 as well as a potent inhibitor of the same). His only other medication has been a baby aspirin. He presents to the Emergency Room with complaints of headache, dizziness, nausea, and reports feeling very anxious and restless. He denies having any hallucinations or dissociations from reality. The attending emergency physician suspects he is suffering from a touch of the flu, however, he is afebrile, his vitals are stable and his antigen screen for Influenza returns as negative. Give the patient's additional report that his symptoms started eight days ago – around the time he was administered his first Abilify Maintenna injection – and have progressively worsened, the emergency physician suspects it might be a drug reaction and calls the on-call consulting psychiatrist. The psychiatrist immediately notices the patient is constantly moving his feet and often gets up to pace. He confirms the patient's symptoms started about forty-eight hours after receiving his injection of Abilify. It is reported that, at one point, the patient had previously been taking Risperdal for approximately four years (primary substrate of CYP2D6). The patient reports that, most recently, his symptoms have been adequately controlled on Latuda 120mg q/day, but reports he started having some re-emergence of auditory hallucinations (Latuda is a primary substrate of CYP3A4). When the dose of Latuda is increased to 140mg daily the patient, soon thereafter, complains of excessive sedation, reporting "I felt kind of sluggish on 120mg daily, but I was just not functioning well on the 140mg dose."

In addition to feeling sedated on the 140mg dose of Latuda, he reports also suffering from nausea "…and I had some of the same restlessness, just not this bad." The psychiatrist discusses options with the patient. The patient is given a 50mg IM dose of Benadryl and within approximately 20 minutes he reports significant improvement in his restlessness (Benadryl is a primary substrate of CYP2D6 and potent inhibitor of the same). He states his nausea, dizziness and headache have also mildly improved. Ninety minutes later the patient's overall symptoms show substantial improvement with resolution of his restlessness and pacing. He reports he feels well enough to be discharged from the ED. The patient is given a prescription for Propanolol 10mg three times daily and an appointment is made to follow-up with his psychiatrist in one week (Propanolol is a primary substrate of CYP2D6). In one week, the patient's psychiatrist observes the patient is doing better, but is still experiencing headache, nausea, and dizziness in addition to mild to moderate symptoms of akathisia. The psychiatrist holds the patient's Fluoxetine dose and orders a Cytochrome P450 genotyping and phenotyping assay, and asks the patient to return in three days. The test results reveal the patient is a normal metabolizer in all three enzyme phenotypes. Upon the patient's return, he reports his symptoms have resolved but is worried about becoming depressed. The psychiatrist starts a trial of Citalopram, and tells the patient to only take Propanolol as needed and only if he feels symptoms of akathisia return (Citalopram is a primary substrate of CYP2C19).

DISCUSSION: This patient's symptoms are common side effects associated with Aripiprazole. In addition to the nausea, dizziness and headache, he presented with classic symptoms of akathisia. The patient's history of suffering akathisia from psychotropic medication in the past – Latuda at 140mg dose – places him at increased risk of suffering future episodes. Abilify Maintenna is predominantly metabolized by the CYP2D6 enzyme and secondarily by CYP3A4. Fluoxetine is primarily metabolized by CYP2D6 but is also a potent CYP2D6 inhibitor (as is Paroxetine and Quinidine). Thus, the patient's actual serum concentration of Aripiprazole and its metabolites, were increased by approximately fifty percent - a marked increase. Interestingly, Propanolol is also primarily metabolized by CYP2D6 and can competitively inhibit the metabolism of Abilify Maintenna. Just as interesting is the fact that Benadryl is a substrate of

CYP2D6 and a potent inhibitor of this enzyme as well. Probably a better choice of treatment for this patient's akathisia would have been an IM dose of Benztropine as this medication does not undergo CYP450 metabolization. Discontinuing Fluoxetine did help resolve most of the patient's symptoms, however, care should also be used while co-administering Propanolol with Abilify. A prudent approach one should consider before starting any long-acting injectable (LAI) medication is to undertake a trial of the oral medication – in this case Abilify oral tablets. Abilify Maintenna comes in a 300mg monthly IM dose and a 400mg monthly IM dose. It is not imprudent, and is quite common, to start a patient on the 400mg dose, unless the patient is elderly or has other risk factors or concerns requiring a reduced dose. For example, in patients taking strong CYP2D6 inhibitors, e.g. Quinidine, Fluoxetine or Paroxetine or CYP3A4 inhibitors (e.g. itraconazole or clarithromycin), the dose of the medication should be cut in half. Thus, a patient can be started on an Ability Maintenna dose of 200mg, but also can be started on 150mg. The same strategy should be followed for patients who are poor CYP2D6 metabolizer phenotypes. The unfortunate result of doing this is that the remainder of the Maintenna vial has to be discarded. For patients taking both strong CYP2D6 and CYP3A4 inhibitors, a quarter of the dose should be used. In most cases, an alternative to either the Abilify Maintenna or the other medications is pursued. For patients simultaneous taking strong CYP3A4 inducers (e.g. Carbamazepine or Rifampin), the dose of Abilify should be doubled. This is generally not recommended unless Abilify and, for example, Carbamazepine are the only combination of psychotropic medications that have been known to have been effective for a patient. Latuda (Lurasidone) is also metabolized mainly via the CYP3A4 enzyme and primarily results in two active metabolizes (ID-14283 and ID-14326) and two inactive metabolites (ID-20219 and ID-20220). In similar rare cases where Latuda is co-administered with Carbamazepine, the dose of Latuda should be increased in increments of 20mg and under close observation. Clinicians should remember that when Latuda is taken with food, serum levels reach maximum concentration than when this medication is taken on an empty stomach. When Latuda is co-administered with moderate CYP3A4 inhibitors, the maximum recommended dose of Latuda is generally 40mg q/day.

Case 13: CYP2D6 Poor Metabolizer
CYP2C19 Normal Metabolizer
CYP2C9 Normal Metabolizer

Key Medications Involved: Atomoxetine, Paroxetine, Citalopram

This patient is a 26 y/o Caucasian female with a diagnosis of Attention-Deficit Hyperactivity Disorder diagnosed approximately three years ago when she started college. She has been treated with Atomoxetine for the past three years with good results (primary CYP2D6 substrate). Her dose has remained at 25 mg daily during this time. The recent death of her mother has triggered symptoms of depression. She reports to her psychiatrist that she has had little interest in school, with her grades significantly suffering. Her appetite has become scant and she has lost about eleven pounds in two months. She has been receiving psychotherapy, however, her symptoms have only worsened over the past four months. Her family history is significant for depression in her older brother who has been treated to remission with Paroxetine (primary CYP2D6 substrate and inhibitor of the same). Given this information, she is started on Paroxetine 20mg at bedtime. Three days later, she presents to the emergency department with chest pain and diaphoresis. She is tachycardic with a heart rate of 117. Her EKG showed tachycardia with non-specific QRS and PR changes. Her toxicology screen and cardiac enzymes returned as negative. She is advised to stop both Paroxetine and Atomoxetine and to follow up with her psychiatrist as soon as possible. Three days later, her psychiatrist orders a Cytochrome P450 genotyping and phenotyping assay. The results indicate the patient is a CYP2D6 poor metabolizer. Atomoxetine is re-started at 25mg daily. After discussing options with the patient, she is started on a trial of Citalopram 10mg q/day. In one week the dose is increased to 20mg q/day. At follow up visits at two weeks and seven weeks respectively, it's noted there has been no significant clinical improvement. The patient requests that Paroxetine be re-started, and it is decided that a lower dose of 5mg be started at bedtime, and Atomoxetine be taken in the mornings. At a follow up visit a week later, the patient reports she is not feeling much better, but has not suffered any side effects. At that visit, it is decided that Atomoxetine be held until she is adequately responding to Paroxetine. Paroxetine is increased to 20mg at bedtime. Two weeks later, the patient comes to her follow up appointment with her sister, who reports she has noticed some improvement in the patient's interest and appetite. The patient reports she "might" be feeling a little better. Four weeks later, she reports she is feeling noticeably better, with improved mood, appetite, energy and interest, but still feels "very depressed" an average of three out of seven days per week. Paroxetine is then increased to 40mg at bedtime. One month later, her symptoms of depression appear to be in partial early remission. At that time she reports she is becoming very frustrated at her inability to maintain her concentration and to complete her school projects on a timely manner. Atomoxetine is re-started at a lower dose of 10mg daily.

Two weeks later, the patient reports she was unable to continue Atomoxetine even at the lowest available dose of10mg daily because she started sweating and experiencing heart palpitations - albeit reportedly less severe than previously experienced. When she discontinued the 10mg Atomoxetine dose, her symptoms resolved. It was decided she would take a medical withdrawal from school and return the next semester. The patient agrees to start cognitive behavioral therapy and to adopt more regular exercise program as part of her treatment for her ADHD. Two months later, she reports her symptoms of depression remain in full remission. She reports still having some crying spells, but associates them with "memories of my mom." She reports she is still struggling with her concentration, but acknowledges "it's better". Two months thereafter, it is decided to taper her off Paroxetine and re-start Atomoxetine (given it has efficacy in both ADHD and secondary efficacy for symptoms of depression). She is re-started on 25mg daily. One month later, the patient reports she feels her symptoms of depression remain in remission and she has re-started school and is doing well.

DISCUSSION: Both Atomoxetine and Paroxetine are principally metabolized by the CYP2D6 enzyme. Paroxetine is an inhibitor of this enzyme. This patient's symptoms were the result of an acute increase in serum Atomoxetine levels from inhibitory effect of Paroxetine on the CYP2D6 enzymes. Atomoxetine levels increase by 3-4 fold when co-administered with Paroxetine with normal CYP2D6 metabolizers as Paroxetine is a CYP2D6 inhibitor. The mean half-life increases from 5.2 to about 10 hours. This patient is a CYP2D6 poor metabolizer. Thus, Atomoxetine levels increased by approximately ten fold or more, causing her acute, and worrisome, symptoms. The decision to start a trial of Citalopram was reasonable as Citalopram is metabolized principally by CYP2C19. Great care should be taken if Atomoxetine and Paroxetine are co-administered.

Case 14: CYP2D6 Poor Metabolizer
CYP2C19 Normal Metabolizer
CYP2C9 Normal Metabolizer

Key Medications Involved: Thorazine, Trazodone, Alprazolam, Ramelteon

This patient is a fifty-one year old Hispanic male with paranoid-type Schizophrenia. He has been stable on a relatively low static dose of Thorazine for a number of years – 50mg twice daily, and an additional 50mg daily as-needed for any break-through auditory hallucinations (Thorazine is extensively metabolized by CYP2D6 and, secondarily, by CYP1A2 and CYP3A4). The patient's records indicate, in the distant past, he has tried Olanzapine, Fluphenazine (Prolixin), Ziprasidone (Geodone) and Haldol, but did not fare very well on any of these. During a routine follow-up visit, the patient reports he has been having difficulty sleeping. He is started on Trazodone 50mg at bedtime (primary CYP2D6 substrate). One week later, his caregiver calls the clinic and reports she took the patient to the emergency room as he had become confused and over-sedated and had fallen twice. The ED physician advised her to discontinue the patient's Trazodone and Thorazine until the he was able to follow-up with his psychiatrist. He does so several days later, accompanied by his caretaker, and is observed to be awake and alert but somewhat paranoid. He reports being bothered by intermittent auditory hallucinations. In addition, he reports he is quite anxious. His urine toxicology screen in the clinic is negative, and a Cytochrome P450 genotyping and phenotyping assay is ordered. The patient is re-started on Thorazine 50mg twice daily and is prescribed Alprazolam 0.5mg twice daily for his anxiety (Alprazolam is a primary substrate of CYP3A4). A follow-up visit is made for three weeks. A few days later, the caretaker calls the clinic reporting the patient is again rather sedated and "a little" confused. She reports his symptoms are not nearly as severe, but she is concerned. She is advised to bring the patient in right away. When they arrive at the psychiatrist's office, the patient reports his auditory hallucinations have nearly resolved and his anxiety is much improved, but reports he "feels drunk". Neurologically, his balance is observed to be modestly impaired and his cognitive processing is rather sluggish. Both his Thorazine and Alprazolam are held and his caretaker is advised to bring him back the next afternoon. At that visit, his sensorium is markedly improved and he has a full level of alertness. He reports his auditory hallucinations are slight but his anxiety has become worse. The result of his pharmacogenetic testing were reviewed as follows: CYP2D6 poor metabolizer, with normal metabolizer phenotype in both the CYP2C19 and CYP2C9 enzymes. The patient is re-started on Thorazine 50mg at bedtime. He and his caretaker are advised to increase the dose to 50mg twice daily in one week only if he is not experiencing any symptoms of sedation. He returns in two weeks and reports overall feeling better, noting his auditory hallucinations have nearly resolved. His caretaker reports she has not noticed any paranoia and "for the most part, he is back to himself". The patient, however, reports he continues to struggle with anxiety and is having difficulty sleeping. After discussing treatment options, he agrees to start psychotherapy to help with his anxiety. To help with sleep, he agrees to start a trial of Ramelteon, as he remembers responding to this in the past (about 50 percent metabolized via CYP1A2 with minor involvement of CYP2C19 and CYP3A4). His caretaker reports he remembers his insurance providing coverage for this medication in the past after a 'prior-authorization' request was submitted. The patient agrees to tentatively follow-up in two weeks, with the caveat that he may return at any time before then should he or his caretaker observe anything concerning. In two weeks the patient returns and reports he is sleeping better, but reports he is still struggling with anxiety. After further exploring the nidus of his symptoms, it is agreed to re-start the as-needed Thorazine dose of 50mg daily. After four sessions of psychotherapy, the patient reports improvement in his anxiety. In addition, he reports the additional as-needed dose of Thorazine is helping his anxiety. He reports he is taking this additional dose, on average, about three times per week.

DISCUSSION: The patient's initial symptoms – over-sedation and confusion – were due to the patient's CYP2D6 poor-metabolizer phenotype status as well as the combined competitive inhibition of the CYP2D6 enzyme by Trazodone and Thorazine. Trazodone is principally metabolized by CYP2D6. Discontinuation of this medication, and holding Thorazine for about 30 hours, would have likely been all that was needed to clear up the patient's symptoms (as the half-life of Thorazine is approximately 30 hours). Thorazine is extensively metabolized by CYP2D6 and, secondarily, by CYP1A2 and CYP3A4. Approximately 35 percent, however, is excreted in the urine unchanged. Given that Alprazolam is a primary substrate of CYP3A4, and the fact that this patient is a CYP2D6 poor metabolizer, both CYP3A4 and CYP3A5 are activated as 'back up' enzymes to CYP2D6. Alprazolam is principally metabolized by the CYP3A4 enzyme. The second round of the patient's sedation and confusion, reportedly milder, were likely due to the combined competitive co-inhibition of CYP3A4 by Thorazine and Alprazolam. Hence, the discontinuation of Alprazolam resolved the patient's symptoms. The use of Ramelteon for sleep disorders is somewhat limited to Circadian shift-work disorder, however, it is not a bad choice here as it is not a controlled substance and is considered a very safe sleep agent. It is a melatonin receptor agonist with no significant toxic dose. It's metabolism consists primarily of oxidation with secondary glucuronidation. It is estimated that less-than half of the drug is metabolized by CYP1A2 with minor involvement of CYP2C9 and CYP3A4, which are not thought to have a clinically significant impact on Ramelteon's metabolization.

Case 15: CYP2D6 Intermediate Metabolizer
CYP3A4 Intermediate Metabolizer
CYP2C19 Normal Metabolizer
CYP2C9 Normal Metabolizer

Key Medications Involved: Fluvoxamine, Modafinil

This patient is a 38 year-old obese Caucasian male with Obsessive-Compulsive Disorder who has been stable on Fluvoxamine (Luvox) 75mg at bedtime and 25mg every morning for several years (Fluvoxamine is primary substrate of CYP2D6 and a potent inhibitor of 3A4). During his last follow-up with his psychiatrist, he complained of excessive daytime sleepiness. His wife, who accompanied him, reported she has noticed for some time that her husband snores loudly and often seems to gasp and wake up "many times" throughout the night. Looking at past records, his weight has gradually increased over the past two years. His BMI is now 45. He does not feel Fluvoxamine is the culprit and reports his primary care physician has ordered Thyroid Function tests as he thinks he may suffer from hypothyroidism. The patient is referred to a sleep medicine specialist. During his next follow-up visit, he reports he completed a polysomnogram which revealed moderate to severe obstructive sleep apnea. He states he recently started using a CPAP machine at night, but reports he still feels tired and sluggish throughout the day. His Fluvoxamine dose is modified to 100mg at bedtime to ensure the 25mg morning dose is not contributing to his daytime fatigue. Three weeks later the patient calls his psychiatrist's office and reports he is experiencing severe anxiety, headache, and nausea. He comes in the next day and reports he was recently started on Modafinil four days ago for excessive daytime sleepiness (approximately 30 percent of Modafinil is metabolized via CYP3A4). His blood pressure is measured as 171/89 (normal blood pressure recorded for this patient had previously been 130-140/80-83. The patient's sleep medicine physician is reached by telephone and agrees the patient should stop the Modafinil. The psychiatrist orders a Cytochrome P450 genotyping and phenotyping assay and the results indicate the patient is a CYP2D6 intermediate metabolizer, a CYP3A4 intermediate metabolizer and a normal metabolizer in the CYP2C19 and CYP2C9 pathways. A week later, the patient returns and reports his symptoms have resolved. His blood pressure at that visit is noted to be much improved at 134/73.

DISCUSSION: This patient's symptoms were caused by a drug-drug-gene interaction between Modafinil and Fluvoxamine. Modafanil is a noradrenergic and histaminergic modulator and increases both central noradrenaline and histamine levels. Modafinil can cause acute hypertension, tachycardia, headache, and nausea. He is a CYP2D6 intermediate metabolizer and a CYP3A4 intermediate metabolizer – which is quite rare in the Caucasian population at a maximum prevalence of 5 percent. Fluvoxamine is primarily metabolized by CYP2D6. It is also a potent CYP3A4 inhibitor. Given the patient's CYP2D6 intermediate metabolizer status, it makes sense that his OCD symptoms are controlled on a relatively low dose of Fluvoxamine (100mg q/day). Metabolism of Modafinil occurs through a non-CYP450 process – hydrolytic deamination, S-oxidation, aromatic ring hydroxylation and glucoronidation – with an estimated 30 percent of this medication metabolized by the CYP3A4 enzyme. Less-than 10 percent of Modafinil is excreted by the kidneys as the unchanged parent compound. In addition to a minor amount of Modafanil being metabolized by CYP3A4, Modafinil is also a strong inducer of this enzyme. Given, however, that the patient is an intermediate CYP3A4 metabolizer, and the fact that Fluvoxamine is a potent inhibitor of this enzyme, the effect on this patient was phenoconversion to a CYP3A4 poor metabolizer – essentially this enzyme became "overwhelmed". The net effect on Modafinil was that it's serum concentration was substantially increased, thereby causing the patient's acute symptoms of severe anxiety, headache, nausea and hypertension. Given the patient is obese, his cardiac risk index is elevated. Knowing his pharmacogenetic profile will provide a modicum of safety when he is started on any new medications.

CONCLUSION

Given the tremendous human and financial effects of adverse drug reactions alone, the use of pharmacogenetic technology should now be considered a viable tool for clinicians. Among the emerging technologies in genetics, pharmacogenetics seems to have emerged as the low hanging fruit, ripe for the picking by the psychiatric medicine practitioner. The emphasis, however, must be on using it as a scalpel...not as a broadsword. Psychiatry has, for too long, suffered from a subjective 'try and see' approach to prescribing medications. This approach has certainly contributed to the tsunami of drug-drug and drug-gene interactions. And considering the fact that psychotropic medications are now the most prescribed drugs in medicine – and far from benign – the emergence of this new and promising technology is auspicious and timely. There is currently underway a transformation in the curriculum of medical schools and residencies which includes, in part, a call to include more education in genetic medicine and, in this vein, pharmacogenetics.[197] For this important science to take root in clinical practice, it will first have to take root in medical education, where change comes slowly. It is apparent, regardless of pace, that change is, nonetheless, inevitable.

The increasingly severe regulatory and legal climate in medicine, coupled with the recommendation by the FDA that this technology be used to guide the prescribing of certain medications, pharmacogenetic technology in psychiatric practice is not only a tool that can help reduce adverse drug reactions and enhance the precision and accuracy of prescribing, but is also an excellent way to reduce individual and collective medical liability. The applied rule of law in medical malpractice clearly places the burden of proof on the practitioner to justify treatment decisions. The employment of empirical tools in the excessively subjective field of psychiatry lends scientific credibility and can be perceived that a clinician has gone above and beyond what most would do to provide an additional ring of safety around treatment decisions. This is especially important if a given treatment involves off-label uses, or doses of medications outside of that recommended by the FDA. Both practices are very common in psychiatry. The subjective trial and error approach to psychiatric treatment that has been its standard operating procedure to date is increasingly burdened with risk. Psychiatrists and other mental health providers are now, more often than not, assumed to be culpable when licensure board complaints and lawsuits arise. They must avail themselves of all useful clinical tools – consistent with the *Reasonable Person Doctrine* – to support their clinical decisions or risk facing sanctions and judgments. The fact that one in five drugs that are approved by the FDA have a pharmacogenetics warning in their label actually creates an obligation to understand the basic tenets of this science and to apply it when warranted. Used properly, and with a trained eye, pharmacogenetic testing can help to substantially mitigate the medico-legal risk of clinical practice.

> *Despite its already established benefits, pharmacogenetics is still a burgeoning field and has yet to meet its potential. It still has to complete the crucial step required of all new modalities in medicine to solidify its credibility – a large double-blind placebo controlled trial.*

Pharmacogenomic technology shows promise on several other fronts. It is allowing us to identify genes with the highest likelihood of predicting efficacy for novel therapeutics and to substantially reduce the size and cost of clinical trials. It has the ability to classify diseases into distinct subcategories which challenges the traditional business model of a 'one-size-fits-all' drug that has been the core of pharmaceutical development. The economic rationale for personalized medicine-driven healthcare decisions is increasingly dependent on the cost savings realized through a given technology. Used appropriately, pharmacogenetics shows excellent promise as a technology to enhance cost effectiveness of both treatment selection and surveillance of response. The data increasingly shows that patients who are phenotypic outliers – such as poor or rapid CYP2D6 metabolizers – have longer hospital stays, suffer more adverse drug reactions, and cost more to treat. Using pharmacogenetic information during utilization reviews as well as to help categorize and streamline the cost of treatment allows a cross pollination of it's utility, and is an additional value to that of it's principal use as a clinical tool. Its impact on disease, over the longer term, has yet to be even realized as this science will surely contribute to fostering economies of scale as well as new biomarkers – both of which are key predictive metrics for major medical breakthroughs.

> *Pharmacogenetics guides the development of drugs in ways that categorize well with certain populations, and any use of such information will need to be carefully implemented to avoid a perception of stigma based on ethnicity or race.*

The greatest clinical benefit of pharmacogenetics to date has clearly been its ability to help more accurately predict an individual's response to a given drug, thereby increasing the success of that treatment and reducing the incidence of side effects. Offering patients personalized genetic information outlining which treatment is more likely to be effective and have fewer side effects can help increase medication adherence, which has been a recurrent challenge in psychiatry since psychotropic medications were formally categorized in the early to mid-twentieth century. A 2013 study by Dolgin and colleagues has been a catalyst for, and has given momentum to, larger studies which are requisite for the wider adoption of pharmacogenetics in clinical practice. Dolgin and his colleagues found that of 1260 test recipients whose psychiatric medications were changed based upon pharmacogenetic testing results, only 33 percent stopped taking their medications at six months compared to 41 percent of matched controls.[198]

Despite its already established benefits, pharmacogenetics is still a burgeoning field and has yet to even come close to its potential as a clinical tool. It still has to complete the crucial step required of all new modalities in medicine seeking wider scientific credibility – a large double-blind placebo-controlled trial. In addition, although there have been laws enacted to protect against the misuse of personal genetic information, such as the Genetic Non-Discrimination Act of 2008, there is still a fair amount of concern about the implications of a technology that simply orbits the controversial topic of genetic profiling, in addition to confidentiality, privacy, and ownership that are involved. Pharmacogenetics guides the development of drugs in ways that categorize well with certain populations, and any use of such information will need to be carefully implemented to avoid a perception of stigma based on ethnicity or race.

The process of phenotype development in pharmacogenetics remains a challenge as its precision and accuracy is directly related to how well the current state of this science is able to make predictions. The wider adoption of pharmacogenetic technology in psychiatric practice, and the development of a central pharmacogenetics database, will no doubt improve its accuracy and effectiveness.

As medicine starts to focus more on wellness rather than disease, pharmacogenetic technology will become more important, and more utilized. More biomarkers, in addition to the CYP450 enzymes, will be employed as more biotechnological and computational tools are used in a coordinated effort to help transform the focus of medicine to a proactive, rather than a reactive, practice. The greater endeavor for this new approach will not be discovery, but the adoption and appropriate utilization of pharmacogenetic technology and new biomarkers in the clinic and at the bedside, where change has always been hard won.

SELECTED PSYCHOTROPIC DRUGS AND THEIR CLINICALLY RELEVANT PHARMACOGENETICS [199]

Drug name (Brand name)	Gene	Clinically Relevant Pharmacogenetics
Aripiprazole (Abilify)	CYP2D6	Poor Metabolizers have approximately 80% increase in Aripiprazole exposure and approximately 30% decrease in exposure to the active metabolite compared to normal metabolizers, resulting in approximately 60% higher exposure to the total active moieties from a given dose of Aripiprazole compared to normal metabolizers. Poor metabolizers have higher exposure to Aripiprazole compared to normal metabolizers; hence, poor metabolizers should have their initial dose reduced by one-half.
Amitriptyline (Elavil)	CYP2D6	Poor metabolizers have higher than expected plasma concentrations of tricyclic antidepressants (TCAs) when given usual doses. Depending on the fraction of drug metabolized by CYP2D6, the increase in plasma concentration may be small or quite large (8-fold increase in plasma AUC of the TCA).
Atomoxetine (Strattera)	CYP2D6	Atomoxetine is metabolized primarily through the CYP2D6 enzymatic pathway. People with reduced activity in this pathway (poor metabolizers) have higher plasma concentrations of Atomoxetine compared to people with normal activity (normal metabolizers). For poor metabolizers, AUC of Atomoxetine is approximately 10-fold and Css max is about 5-fold greater than in normal metabolizers. Dose adjustment may be necessary.
Citalopram (Celexa)	CYP2C19	In CYP2C19 poor metabolizers, Citalopram steady state Cmax and AUC was increased by 68% and 107%, respectively. 20 mg/day is the maximum recommended dose in CYP2C19 poor metabolizers due to the risk of QT prolongation.

Clomipramine (Anafranil)	CYP2D6	Poor metabolizers have higher than expected plasma concentrations of tricyclic antidepressants (TCAs) when given usual doses. Depending on the fraction of drug metabolized by CYP2D6, the increase in plasma concentration may be small or quite large (8-fold increase in plasma AUC of the TCA).
Clozapine (Clozaril)	CYP2D6	Dose reduction may be necessary in patients who are CYP2D6 poor metabolizers. Clozapine concentrations may be increased in these patients, because Clozapine is almost completely metabolized and then excreted.
Desipramine (Norpramin)	CYP2D6	Poor metabolizers have higher than expected plasma concentrations of tricyclic antidepressants (TCAs) when given usual doses. Depending on the fraction of drug metabolized by CYP2D6, the increase in plasma concentration may be small or quite large (8-fold increase in plasma AUC of the TCA).
Doxepin (Silenor)	CYP2D6 CYP2C19	Poor metabolizers of CYP2C19 and CYP2D6 may have higher Doxepin plasma levels than normal subjects.
Fluvoxamine (Luvox CR)	CYP2D6	Caution is indicated in patients known to have reduced levels of CYP2D6 activity and those receiving concomitant drugs known to inhibit this cytochrome P450 isoenzyme.
Iloperidone (Fanapt)	CYP2D6	Iloperidone dose should be reduced by one-half for poor metabolizers of CYP2D6.
Imipramine (Tofranil-PM)	CYP2D6	Poor metabolizers have higher than expected plasma concentrations of tricyclic antidepressants (TCAs) when given usual doses. Depending on the fraction of drug metabolized by CYP2D6, the increase in plasma concentration may be small or quite large (8-fold increase in plasma AUC of the TCA).

Nortriptyline (Pamelor)	CYP2D6	Poor metabolizers have higher than expected plasma concentrations of tricyclic antidepressants (TCAs) when given usual doses. Depending on the fraction of drug metabolized by CYP2D6, the increase in plasma concentration may be small or quite large (8-fold increase in plasma AUC of the TCA).
Perphenazine (Trilafon)	CYP2D6	CYP2D6 poor metabolizers will metabolize Perphenazine more slowly and will experience higher concentrations compared with normal or "normal" metabolizers.
Pimozide (Orap)	CYP2D6	Individuals with genetic variations resulting in poor CYP2D6 metabolism (approximately 5 to 10% of the population) exhibit higher Pimozide concentrations than normal CYP2D6 metabolizers. Alternative dosing strategies are recommended in patients who are genetically poor CYP2D6 metabolizers.
Protriptyline (Vivactil)	CYP2D6	Poor metabolizers have higher than expected plasma concentrations of tricyclic antidepressants (TCAs) when given usual doses. Depending on the fraction of drug metabolized by CYP2D6, the increase in plasma concentration may be small or quite large (8-fold increase in plasma AUC of the TCA).
Thioridazine (Mellaril)		Caution in patients with reduced CYP2D6 isozyme activity. Drugs which inhibit this isozyme, and certain other drugs appear to appreciably inhibit the metabolism of Thioridazine. The resulting elevated levels of thioridazine would be expected to augment the prolongation of the QTc interval associated with Thioridazine and may increase the risk of serious, potentially fatal, cardiac arrhythmias, such as Torsades de pointes type arrhythmias.
Trimipramine (Surmontil)	CYP2D6	Poor metabolizers have higher than expected plasma concentrations of tricyclic antidepressants (TCAs) when given usual doses. Depending on the fraction of drug metabolized by CYP2D6, the increase in plasma concentration may be small or quite large (8-fold increase in plasma AUC of the TCA).

The table below describes some of the web resources, including their names, web links, main contents, and an extra rating column.[200 201 202 203 204] Zhang et al rated these web sources based on several factors including their relations to pharmacogenomics, their data sizes, the number and usefulness of the applications provided on the website, and the overall user experience.

MAJOR WEB SOURCES FOR PHARMACOGENOMICS

Name	Link	Main features
PharmGKB	http://www.pharmgkb.org/	Natural Language Processing and manual curation variants, associations between variants and drugs, drug-centered pathways, genotype-based pharmacogenomic summaries
CPIC	http://www.pharmgkb.org/page/cpic/	Detailed gene/drug clinical practice guidelines, drug dosing guidelines
DrugBank	http://www.drugbank.ca/	Drug-based information, drug pharmacogenomics, drug/food interaction, metabolic enzymes, Quantitative Structure Activity Relationship, ADME data
SCAN	http://www.scandb.org/	SNP annotation, GWAS analysis tool
PACdb	http://www.pacdb.org/	Pharmacology-related information including genotypes, gene expressions, and pharmacological data obtained via Lymphoblastoid cell line
Human Cytochrome P450 Allele Nomenclature database	http://www.cypalleles.ki.se/	CYP450 alleles, CYP450 isoforms, relationship between genotype and phenotype
Cytochrome P450 Drug Interaction Table	http://medicine.iupui.edu/clinpharm/ddis/clinical-table/	Drug and CYP450 isoform interaction
FDA's pharmacogenetic website	http://www.fda.gov/drugs/scienceresearch/researchareas/pharmacogenetics/ucm083378.html	Clinical response and drug exposure variability, dosing recommendation according to genotypes, drug mechanisms, germline or somatic gene variant biomarkers

BIBLIOGRAPHY

Ahmad A, Mast MR, Nijpels G, Elders PJ, Dekker JM, Hugtenburg JG. Identification of drug-related problems of elderly patients discharged from hospital. *Patient Prefer Adherence.* 2014;8:155-65.

Aizenberg D, Gur S, Zemishlany Z, et al. Mianserin, a 5-HT2a/2c and alpha 2 antagonist, in the treatment of sexual dysfunction induced by serotonin reuptake inhibitors. *Clin Neuropharmacol.* 20(3):210-214 (1997).

Alagoz O, Durham D, Kasirajan K. (2015) Cost Effectiveness of One-Time Genetic Testing to Minimize Lifetime Adverse Drug Reactions. *The Pharmacogenomics Journal.* 19 May 2015 Issue. 39:1-8.

Ashton AK, Hamer R, Rosen R. Serotonin reuptake inhibitor-induced sexual dysfunction and its treatment: A large-scale retrospective study of 596 psychiatric outpatients. *J Sex Marital Ther.* 23(3):165-175 (1997).

Balogh S, Hendricks SE, Kang J. Treatment of fluoxetine-induced anorgasmia with amantadine. *J Clin Psychiatry.* 53:212-213 (1992).

Balon R. Intermittent amantadine for fluoxetine-induced anorgasmia. *J Sex Marital Ther.* 22: 290-292 (1996).

Beijer HJ, de Blaey CJ. Hospitalizations caused by adverse drug reactions (ADR): a meta-analysis of observational studies. *Pharm World Sci.* 2002 Apr;24(2):46-54.

Berenbeim DM. Polypharmacy: overdosing on good intentions. *Manag Care Q.* 2002;10(3):1-5

Birdwell KA, Decker B, Barbarino JM, et al. : Clinical pharmacogenetics implementation consortium (CPIC) guidelines for CYP3A5 genotype and tacrolimus dosing. *Clin Pharmacol Ther.* 2015 Jul;98(1):19-24.

Biskupiak J, Biltaji E, Bress A, Ye X, Unni S, Newman R, Ashcraft A, Mamiya T, Brixner D. Cost-consequence analysis for pharmacogenetic testing in an Elderly Population. *Journal of Managed Care & Specialty Pharmacy.* Oct 2015. Vol.21, No. 10-a: S81.

Brixner D, Biltaji E, Bress A, Unni S, Ye X, Mamiya T, Ashcraft A, Biskupiak J. The effect of pharmacogenetic profiling with a clinical decision support tool on healthcare resource utilization and estimated costs in the elderly exposed to polypharmacy. *Journal of Medical Economics.* 19(3):213-28 (2016).

Biskupiak J, Unni S, Thirumaran RK, Biltaji E, Bress A, Ye X, Ashcraft K, Brixner D. Impact of pharmacogenetics with integrated clinical decision support on healthcare utilization and costs in the elderly receiving polypharmacy: Report update. (Unpublished Data)

Bozina N, Bradamante V, Lovric M. Genetic polymorphism of metabolic enzymes P450 (CYP) as a susceptibility factor for drug response, toxicity, and cancer risk. *Arh Hig Rada Toksikol.* 2009;60(2):217-42.

Cai WM, Nikoloff DM, Pan RM, de Leon J, Fanti P, Fairchild M et al. CYP2D6 genetic variation in healthy adults and psychiatric African-American subjects: implications for clinical practice and genetic testing. *Pharmacogenomics J.* 2006 Sep-Oct;6(5):343-50.

Callaghan JT, Bergstrom RF, Ptak LR, Beasley CM. Olanzapine: pharmacokinetic and pharmacodynamic profile. *Clin. Pharmacokinet*. 177-93 (1999).

Center for Devices and Radiologic Health, et.al. US Food and Drug Administration, Guidance for Industry and FDA Staff: Pharmacogenetic Tests and Geneitc Tests for Heritable Markers 3 (2007).

Chou, WH, Yan FX, et.al. Extension of a pilot study: impact from the cytochrome P450 2D6 polymorphism on outcome and costs associated with severe mental illness. *J Clin Psychopharmacol*. 20(2):246-51 (April 2000).

Classen DC, Pestotnik SL, Evans RS, et al. Adverse drug events in hospitalized patients. *JAMA*. 277(4):301-6 (1997).

Cohen AJ. Gingko biloba for drug-induced sexual dysfunction. Abstracts of the Annual Meeting of the American Psychiatric Association, San Diego, Calif. p 15 (1997).

Crews KR, Gaedigk A, Dunnenberger HM, Leeder JS et al. Clinical Pharmacogenetics Implementation Consortium guidelines for cytochrome P450 2D6 genotype and codeine therapy: 2014 update *Clin Pharmacol Ther*. 2014 Apr;95(4):376-82.

Cullen DJ, Bates DW, Small SD, et al. The incident reporting system does not detect adverse drug events: A problem for quality improvement. *Journal on Quality Improvement*. 21(10):541-8 (1995).

Daly AK. Significance of the minor cytochrome P450 3A isoforms. *Clin Pharmacokinet*. 45(1):13-31 (2006).

de Leon J, Susce MT, Johnson M, Hardin M, Maw L, Shao A et al. DNA Microarray Technology in the Clinical Environment: The AmpliChip CYP450 Test for CYP2D6 and CYP2C19 Genotyping. *CNS Spectr*. 2009;14(1):19-34 de Montello, ed. *Cytochrome P450 Structure, Mechanism and Biochemitry*, 3rd Ed. Kluwer Academic/Plenum Publishers (2005).

Desta Z, Zhao X, Shin JG, Flockhart DA. Clinical significance of the cytochrome P450 2C19 genetic polymorphism. *Clin Pharmacokinet*. 2002;41(12):913-58.

Dolgin, Ellie. Pharmacogenetic tests yield bonus benefit: better drug adherence. *Nature Medicine*. 19:11, 1354-5 (November 2013).

Doucet J, Chassagne P, Trivalle C, Landrin I, Pauty MD, Kadri N, et al. Drug-drug interactions related to hospital admissions in older adults - a prospective study of 1000 patients. *American Geriatrics Society*. 1996;44(8).

Dreifus C. A conversation with Arno Motulsky: A Genetics Pioneer Sees a Bright Future, Cautiously. *The New York Times* (April 29, 2008). http://www.nytimes.com/2008/04/29/science

Durham, D. *Utilizing Pharmacogenetic Testing in Psychiatry – data from the New Mexico cohort*. Healthshire Publishing (2013). http://www.healthshire.com/utilizing-pharmacogenetic-testing-in-psychiatry-the-time-is-now%e2%80%a8/

Elens L, van Gelder T, Hesselink DA, Haufroid V, van Schaik RH. CYP3A4*22: promising newly identified CYP3A4 variant allege for personalizing pharmacotherapy. *Pharmacogenomics*. 2013:14(1): 47-62.

Evans WE, Relling RV: Pharmacogenomics: translating functional genomics into rational therapeutics. *Science* 1999;486:487-491.

Floyd MD, Gervasini G, Masica Al, et. al. Genotyp-phenotyp associations for common CYP3A4 and CYP3A5 variants in the basal and induced metabolism of midazolam in European and African-American men and women. *Pharmacogenetics.* 13(10:595-606 (October, 2003).

Frye, R.F., Chapter 3: Pharmacogenetics of Oxidative Drug Metabolism and its clinical applications. *Pharmacogenomics:Applications to Patient Care.* Washington, D.C: American College of Clinical Pharmacy (2009).

Gamazon ER, Duan S, Zhang W, Huang RS, Kistner EO, Dolan ME, et al. PACdb: a database for cell-based pharmacogenomics. *Pharmacogenet Genomics* 2010;20:269–73.

Gamazon ER, Huang RS, Cox NJ. SCAN: a systems biology approach to pharmacogenomic discovery. *Methods Mol Biol* 2013;1015:213–24.

Garay MLG. The road from next-generation sequencing to personalized medicine. *Personalized Medicine* (2014) 11 (5), 523-544.

Goldbloom DS, Kennedy SH. Adverse interaction of fluoxetine and cyproheptadine in two patients with bulimia nervosa. *Clin Psychiatry.* 52:261-262 (1991).

Goodall, D.S. The Molecular Perspective: Cytochrome P450. *The Oncologist.* vol. 6 no. 2; p 205-206 (April 2001).

Gross MD. Reversal by bethanechol of sexual dysfunction caused by anticholinergic antidepressants. *Am J Psychiatry.* 139:1193-1194 (1982).

Gurwitz D, Lunshof JE, Dedoussis G *et al.*: Pharmacogenomics education: International Society of Pharmacogenomics recommendations for medical, pharmaceutical, and health schools deans of education. *Pharmacogenomics J.* 5, 221–225 (2005).

Hall-Flavin DK, Winner JG, Allen JD, Jordan JJ, Nesheim RS, Snyder KA, et al. Using a pharmacogenomic algorithm to guide the treatment of depression. *Transl Psychiatry.* 2:e172 (2012).

Hall-Flavin DK, Winner JG, Allen JD, Carhart JM, Proctor B, Snyder KA, et al. Utility of integrated pharmacogenomic testing to support the treatment of major depressive disorder in a psychiatric outpatient setting. *Pharmacogenetics and genomics.* 23(10):535-48. (2013).

Hamburg MA, Collins FS. The path to personalized medicine. *N Engl J Med.* 2010; 363(4):301-4.

He P, Court MH, Greenblatt DJ, Von Moltke LL. Genotype-phenotype associations of cytochrome P450 3A4 and 3A5 polymorphism clearance in vivo. *Clin Pharmacaol Ther*; 77(5): 373-87 (May 2005).

Healy D, Herxheimer A, Menkes DB: Antidepressants and violence: problems at the interface of medicine and law. *PloS* 3, 1478–1487 (2006).

Healy, M. Doctors Untrained to Utilize Genetic Testing. *Los Angeles Times* (Oct 24, 2009).

Hein, D.W., Boukouvala, S., Grant, D.M., Minchin, R.F. & Sim, E. Changes in consensus arylamine N-acetyltransferase gene nomenclature. *Pharmacogenetics and genomics* 18, 367-8 (2008).

Higgins A, Nash M, Lynch A. Antidepressant-associated sexual dysfunction: impact, effects, and treatment. *Drug Health & Patient Safety.* 2010; 2: 141–150 (September 9, 2010).

Ho PC, Abbott FS, et al. Influence of CYP2C9 genotypes on the formation of a hepatotoxic metabolite of valproic acid in human liver microsomes. *Pharmacogenomic J.* 3(6):335-42 (2003).

Hocum B, White JR, Heck J, Thirumaran RK, Moyer N, Newman R & Ashcraft K. Cytochrome P450 gene testing & drug interaction analysis in mixed-race, U.S. patients referred for PGx testing. *American Journal of Health-System Pharmacy.* 73(2):61-7 (January 2016).

Hohl CM, Dankoff J, Colacone A, Afilalo M. Polypharmacy, adverse drug-related events, and potential adverse drug interactions in elderly patients presenting to an emergency department. *Ann Emerg Med.* 2001;38(6):666-671.

Hollander E, McCarley A. Yohimbine treatment of sexual side effects induced by serotonin reuptake blockers. *J Clin Psychiatry.* 53(6):207-209 (1992).

Horn, J, Hansten, D. Get to Know an Enzyme: CYP2C9. *Pharmacy Times.* March (2008) Publ http://www.pharmacytimes.com/publications/issue/2008/2008-03/2008-03-8462#sthash.iZ8anpjl.dpuf

Hukkanen, A. Jacob, P. Benowitz, N. Metabolism and Disposition Kinetics of Nicotine. *Pharmacological Reviews.* Vol. 57, No. 1; 79-115. March

Ingelman-Sundberg M. Genetic polymorphisms of cytochrome P450 2D6 (CYP2D6): clinical consequences, evolutionary aspects and functional diversity. Karolinska Institute. *The Pharmacogenomics Journal.* 5, 6–13 (October 2004).

Jacobsen FM. Fluoxetine-induced sexual dysfunction and an open trial of yohimbine. *J Clin Psychiatry.* 53:119-122 (1992).

Kalman LV., et.al Pharmacogenetic allele nomenclature: International workgroup recommendations for test result reporting. *Clinical Pharmacology & Therapeutics. 99(2):172-85 (February 2016).*

Kalow W. Pharmacogenetics – the Heredity and the Response to Drugs. *Journ. Pharmaceu. Sc.* Vol. 52. Issue 2. P. 208 (February 1963).

Kapelyukh Y, Paine MJ, Marechal JD, Sutcliffe MJ, Wolf CR, Roberts GC. Multiple substrate binding by cytochrome P450 3A4: estimation of the number of bound substrate molecules. *Drug Metab Dispos.* 2008;36(10):2136-44.

Katz RJ, Rosenthal M. Adverse interaction of cyproheptadine with serotonergic antidepressants. *J Clin Psychiatry.* 55:314-315 (1994).

Kearns GL, Leeder JS, Gaedigk A.Impact of the CYP2C19*17 allele on the pharmacokinetics of omeprazole and pantoprazole in children: evidence for a differential effect. *Drug Metab Dispos.* 2010 Jun;38(6):894-7.

Kirchheiner J, Nickchen K, Bauer M, et al. Pharmacogenetics of antidepressants and antipsychotics: the contribution of allelic variations to the phenotype of drug response. *Mol Psychiatry.* 2004;9:442–473.

Kitzmiller JP1, Groen DK, Phelps MA, Sadee W. Pharmacogenomic testing: relevance in medical practice: why drugs work in some patients but not in others. *Cleve Clin J Med.* 2011 Apr;78(4):243-57

Kiyotani K, Shimizu M, Kumai T, Kamataki T, Kobayashi S, Yamazaki H. Limited effects of frequent CYP2D6*36-*10 tandem duplication allele on in vivo dextromethorphan metabolism in a Japanese population. *Eur J Clin Pharmacol.* 2010 Oct;66(10):1065-8.

Kraupl TF. Loss of libido in depression. *BMJ.* 1:305 (1972).

Kupfer A, Preisig, R. Pharmacogenetics of mephenytoin: a new drug hydroxylation polymorphism in man. *Eur J Clin Pharmacol.* 26: 753-759 (1984).

Lamba JK, Lin YS, Schuetz EG, Thummel KE. Genetic contribution to variable human CYP3A-mediated metabolism. *Adv Drug Deliv Rev.* 54(10):1271-94 (November 18, 2002).

Larkin v. Pfizer, Inc., 152 S.W.3d 758, 763-64 (Ky. 2004).

Law V, Knox C, Djoumbou Y, Jewison T, Guo AC, Liu Y, et al. DrugBank 4.0: shedding new light on drug metabolism. *Nucleic Acids Res* 2014;42:D1091–7.

Lazarou J, Pomeranz BH, Corey PN. Incidence of adverse drug reactions in hospitalized pateints: a meta-analysis of prospective studies. *JAMA.* 279(15):1200-1205 (1998).

Leeder JS, Developmental Aspects of Drug Metabolism in Children. Therapeutic Innovation & Regulatory Science Oct 1996 vol. 30 no. 4 1135-1143.

Leeder JS, Kearns GL.Pharmacogenetics in pediatrics. Implications for practice. *Pediatr Clin North Am.* 1997 Feb;44(1):55-77.

Lindley CM, Tully MP, Paramsothy V, Tallis RC. Inappropriate Medication is a Major Cause of Adverse Drug Reactions in Elderly Patients. *Age Ageing.* 1992;21:294-300.

Li-Wan-Po A., Girard T., et. al. Pharmacogenetics of CYP2C19: functional and clinical implications of a new variant CYP2C19*17. *Br J Clin Pharmacol.* 69(3): 222–230 (March 2010).

Lucas RA, Gilfillan DJ, Bergstrom RF. A pharmacokinetic interaction between carbamazepine and olanzapine: observations on possible mechanism. *Eur J Clin Pharmacol.* 54:639-43 (1998).

Lucire Y, Crotty C. Antidepressant-induced akathisia-related homicides associated with diminishing mutations in metabolizing genes of the CYP450 family. *Pharmgenomics Pers Med.* 2011;4:65-81.

Lyon E, Foster JG, Palomaki GE, Pratt VM, Reynolds K, Sabato MF et al. Laboratory testing of CYP2D6 alleles in relation to tamoxifen therapy. *Genet Med.* 2012;14(12):990-1000.

Lyon, ER. A review of the effects of nicotine on schizophrenia and antipsychotic medications. *Psychatr. Serv.* 50(10): 1346-50. (October 1999).

Ma Q, Lu AY. The challenges of dealing with promiscuous drug-metabolizing enzymes, receptors and transporters. *Curr Drug Metab.* 9:374–383 (2008).

Mäenpää J, Wrighton S, Bergstrom R, Cerimele B, Tatum D, Hatcher B, et al. Pharmacokinetic and pharmacodynamic interactions between fluvoxamine and olanzapine. *Clin Pharmacol Ther.* 61:225 (1997).

Man M, Farmen M, Dumaual C, Teng CH, Moser B, Irie S et al. Genetic variation in metabolizing enzyme and transporter genes: comprehensive assessment in 3 major East Asian subpopulations with comparison to Caucasians and Africans. *J Clin Pharmacol.* 2010 Aug;50(8):929-40.

McCormick S, Olin J, Brotman AW. Reversal of fluoxetine-induced anorgasmia by cyproheptadine in two patients. *J Clin Psychiatry.* 51:383-384 (1990).

Mejin M, Tiong WN, Lai LYH, Tiong LL, Bujang AM, Hwang SS et al. CYP2C19 genotypes and their impact on clopidogrel responsiveness in percuteneous coronary intervention. *Int J Clin Pharm.* 2013;35:621-28.

Morales A, Condra M, Owen JA, et al: Is yohimbine effective in the treatment of organic impotence? Results of a controlled trial. *J Urol.* 137:1168-1172 (1987).

Motulsky AG. Drug reactions enzymes, and biochemical genetics. *J Am Med Assoc.* 165:835–837. (1957).

Mrazek, D. *Clinical Implementation of Psychiatric Pharmacogenomic Testing: characterizing and displaying genetic variants for clinical action.* Mayo Clinic. (December 2, 2011).

Mrazek, D. *Psychiatric Pharmacogenomics.* Oxford Un. Press (2011).

Mullis, KF, Faloona F, Scharf S, Saiki R, Horn G, and Erlich H. *Specific enzymatic amplification of DNA in vitro: the polymerase chain reaction.* Cold Spring Harbor Symposium in Quantitative Biology, 51:263–273 (1986).

Nebert DW, Zhang G, Vesell ES et. al. From human genetics and genomics to pharmacogenetics and pharmacogenomics: past lessons, future directions. *Drug Metab Rev.* 40:187–224 (2008).

Niwa T, Murayama N, and Yamazaki, H. Comparison of the Contributions of Cytochromes P450 3A4 and 3A5 in Drug Oxidation Rates and Substrate Inhibition. *Journal of Health Science.* 56:239-256 (2010).

Norden MJ. Buspirone treatment of sexual dysfunction associated with selective serotonin reuptake inhibitors. *Depression.* 2:109-112 (1994).

Olesen OV, Linnet K. Olanzapine serum concentrations in psychiatric patients given standard doses: the influence of co-medication. *Ther Drug Metab.* 21:87-90 (1999).

Paine MF, Hart HL, Ludington SS, Haining RL, Rettie AE, Zeldin DC. The human intestinal cytochrome P450 "pie". *Drug Metab Dispos.* 2006 May;34(5):880-6.

Paulozzi, L. Div of Unintentional Injury Prevention; Annest J. Office of Statistics and Programming, National Center for Injury Prevention and Control. United States Centers for Disease Control. *Unintentional Poisoning Deaths – United States 1999 – 2004.* (2005).

Perera V, Gross AS, Polasek TM, Qin Y, Rao G, Forrest A, et al. Considering CYP1A2 phenotype and genotype for optimizing the dose of olanzapine in the management of schizophrenia. *Expert opinion on drug metabolism & toxicology.* 2013;9(9):1115-37.

Perez v. Wyeth Labs, Inc., 734 A.2d 1245, 1255-56 (N.J. 1999).

Personalized Medicine Coalition. *The Case for Personalized Medicine.* 4th Edition 2014.

Phillips KA, Veenstra, DL, Oren, E, et al. Potential role of pharma-cogenomics in reducing adverse drug reactions: a systematic review. *JAMA.* 286:2270 – 2279 (2001).

Preissner SC, Hoffmann MF, Preissner R, Dunkel M, Gewiess A and Preissner S. Polymorphic Cytochrome P450 Enzymes (CYPs) and Their Role in Personalized Therapy. *PLoS One.* 2013; 8(12): e82562.

Preskorn SH, Kane CP, Lobello K, et al. Cytochrome P450 2D6 phenoconversion is common in patients being treated for depression: implications for personalized medicine. *J Clin Psychiatry.* 2013;74(6):614-621.

Price J, Grunhaus LJ: Treatment of clomipramine-induced anorgasmia with yohimbine: A case report. *J Clin Psychiatry.* 51:32-33 (1990).

Provenzani A, Notarbartolo M, Labbozzetta M, Poma P, Vizzini G, Salis P et al.: Influence of CYP3A5 and ABCB1 gene polymorphisms and other factors on tacrolimus dosing in Caucasian liver and kidney transplant patients. *Int J Mol Med.* 2011 Dec;28(6):1093-102.

Quaranta S, Chevalier D, Allorge D, Lo-Guidice JM, et. al. Ethnic differences in the distribution of CYP3A5 gene polymorphisms. *Xenobiotica.* 36(12):1191-1200 (2006).

Ravyn D. et. al CYP450 pharmacogenetic treatment strategies for antipsychotics: A review of the evidence. *Schizophr Res* 2013; 149:3.

Redick TP. Twenty-First Century Toxicogenomics Meets Twentieth Mass Tort Precedent: Is There a Duty to Warn of a "Hypothetical" Harm to an Eggshell Gene? *Washburn Law J.* 547, 667 (2003).

Relling, MV, Klein TE. CPIC: Clinical Pharmacogenetics Implementation Consortium of the Pharmacogenomics Research Network. *Clinical Pharmacology and Therapeutics.* Vol.89. No.3. (March 2011).

Rettie AE, Jones JP. Clinical and Toxicological Relevance of CYP2C9: Drug-Drug Interactions and Pharmacogenetics. *Annu. Rev. Pharmacol. Toxicol.* 45:477-94 (2005).

Reynolds RD. Sertraline-induced anorgasmia treated with intermittent nefazodone. *J Clin Psychiatry.* 58:89 (1997).

Richards S et al. Standards and guidelines for the interpretation of sequence variants: a joint consensus recommendation of the American College of Medical Genetics and Genomics and the Association for Molecular Pathology. *Genetics in medicine.* 2015; 17 (5). 405 - 424.

Ring BJ, Catlow J, Lindsay TJ, Gillespie T, Roskos LK, Cerimele BJ, et al. Identification of the human cytochromes P450 responsible for the in vitro formation of the major oxidative metabolites of the antipsychotic agent olanzapine. *J Pharmacol Exp Ther* 276:658-66 (1996).

Robarge, J.D., Li, L., Desta, Z., Nguyen, A. & Flockhart, D.A. The star-allele nomenclature: retooling for translational genomics. *Clinical pharmacology and therapeutics* 82, 244-8 (2007).

Robert, J., Le Morvan, V., Giovannetti, E., Peters, G.J. & EORTC, P.G.o. On the use of pharmacogenetics in cancer treatment and clinical trials. *European journal of cancer* 50, 2532-43 (2014).

Rosemary J, Adithan C. The Pharmacogenetics of CYP2C9 and CYP2C19: Ethnic Variation and Clinical Significance. *Current Clinical Pharmacology.* 2007;2:93-109.

Roy JN, Lajoie J, Zijenah LS, Barama A, et. al. CYP3A5 genetic polymorphisms in different ethnic populations. *Drug Metab Dispos.* 33(7):884-887 (2005).

Ruano G, Szarek B, Villagra D, Gorowski K, et. Al. Length of psychiatric hospitalization is correlated with CYP2D6 functional status in inpatients with major depressive disorder. *Biomarkers Med.* 7(3), 429-439 (2013).

Runde I, et. al., 2011, *Translational Psychiatry.*

Sallee FR, DeVane CL, Ferrell RE: Fluoxetine-related death in a child with cytochrome P-450 2D6 genetic deficiency. *J. Child. Adolesc. Psychopharmacol.* 10, 327–334 (2000).

Samer CF, Lorenzini KI, Rollason V, Daali Y, Desmeules JA. Applications of CYP450 testing in the clinical setting. *Molecular diagnosis & therapy.* 2013;17(3):165-84.

Schadt, E. Molecular Networks as Sensors and Drivers of Common Human Diseases. 461 *Nature* 218 (2001).

Scordo M, Aklillu E, et al. Genetic polymorphism of cytochrome P450 2C9 in a Caucasian and a black African population. *Br J Clin Pharmacol.* 52(4): 447–450 (October 2001).

Scott SA, Khasawneh R, Peter I, Kornreich R, Desnick RJ. Combined CYP2C9, VKORC1 and CYP4F2 frequencies among racial and ethnic groups. *Pharmacogenomics.* 2010;11(6):781-91.

Segraves RT. Effects of psychotropic drugs on human erection and ejaculation. *Arch Gen Psychiatry.* 46:275-284 (1989).

Shimada T, Yamazaki H, Mimura M, Inui Y, Guengerich FP. Interindividual variations in human liver cytochrome P-450 enzymes involved in the oxidation of drugs, carcinogens and toxic chemicals: studies with liver microsomes of 30 Japanese and 30 Caucasians. *J Pharmacol Exp Ther.* 1994 Jul;270(1):414-23.

Shrivastava RK, Shrivastava S, Overweg N, et al: Amantadine in the treatment of sexual dysfunction associated with selective serotonin reuptake inhibitors. *J Clin Psychopharmacol.* 15:83-84 (1993).

Sim SC, Risinger C, Dahl ML, Aklillu E, Christensen M, Bertilsson L et al. A common novel CYP2C19 gene variant causes ultrarapid drug metabolism relevant for the drug response to proton pump inhibitors and antidepressants. *Clin Pharmacol Ther.* 2006;79:103-13.

Simon T, Verstuyft C, Mary-Krause M, Quteineh L, Drouet E, Méneveau N, et al. Genetic Determinants of Response to Clopidogrel and Cardiovascular Events. *NEJM.* 2009;360(4):363-75.

Sjöqvist, F, et. Al. Plasma level of monomethylated tricyclic antidepressants and side effects in man. *Excepta Medica.* International Congress Series. No 145; p 246-257.

Sorscher SM, Dilsaver SC. Antidepressant-induced sexual dysfunction in men: Due to cholinergic blockade? *J Clin Psychopharmacol.* 6:53-55 (1986).

Surendiran A, Pradhan SC, Adithan C. Role of pharmacogenomics in drug discovery and development. *Indian J Pharmacol.* 2008 Aug; 40(4): 137–143.

Thorn CF, Aklillu E, Klein TE, Altman RB. PharmGKB summary: very important pharmacogene information for CYP1A2. *Pharmacogenetics and genomics.* 22(1):73-7 (2012).

Timmer CJ, Sitsen JM, Delbressine LP. Clinical Pharmacokinetics of Mirtazepine. *Clinical Pharmacokinetics.* June; 38(6) 461-74 (2000).

Tulner LR, Frankfort SV, et.al. Drug-drug interactions in a geriatric outpatient cohort: prevalence and relevance. *Drugs Aging.* 25(4):343-355 (2008).

Van Booven D, Marsh S, McLeod H, Carrillo MW, Sangkuhl K, Klein TE, Altman RB: Cytochrome P450 2C9-CYP2C9. *Pharmacogenetics and Genomics*. 2010 Apr;20(4):277-81.

Van Schaik, R.H., van der Heiden, I.P., van den Anker, J.N. & Lindemans, J. CYP3A5 variant allele frequencies in Dutch Caucasians. *Clinical chemistry* 2002; 48, 1668-7.

Bit P, Mamiya T, Oesterheld J. How common are drug and gene interactions? Prevalence in a sample of 1143 patients with CYP2C9, CYP2C19 and CYP2D6 genotyping. *Pharmacogenomics* (2014) 15(5), 655–665

Vesell ES, Page JG. Genetic control of drug levels in man: phenylbutazone. *Science*. 159:1479–1480 (1968).

Villagra, D. et al. Novel drug metabolism indices for pharmacogenetic functional status based on combinatory genotyping of CYP2C9, CYP2C19 and CYP2D6 genes. *Biomarkers in medicine* 5, 427-438 (2011).

Vogel F. Moderne probleme der humangenetik. *Ergeb Inn Med Kinderheilkd.* 12:52–125 (1959).

Wang D, Guo Y, Wrighton SA, et al: Intronic polymorphism in CYP3A4 affects hepatic expression and response to statin drugs. *Pharmacogenomics J*;11:274-286 (2011).

Wang G, Lei HP, Li Z, Tan ZR, Guo D, Fan L, Chen Y, Hu DL, Wang D, Zhou HH. The CYP2C19 ultra-rapid metabolizer genotype influences the pharmacokinetics of voriconazole in healthy male volunteers. *Eur J Clin Pharmacol.* 65:281–5 (2009).

Watson JD, Crick FH. Molecular structure of nucleic acids; a structure for deoxyribose nucleic acid. *Nature* 171 (4356): 737–738. (April 1953).

Weinshilboum, R. Sladek, SL. Mercaptopurine pharmacogenetics: monogenic inheritance of erythrocyte thiopurine methyltransferase activity. *Am J Hum Genet.* 32(5):651-62 (September 1980).

Wen X, Wang JS, et al. In vitro evaluation of valproic acid as an inhibitor of human cytochrome P450 isoforms: preferential inhibition of cytochrome P450 2C9 (CYP2C9). *British J. Clin. Pharmacol.* Nov;52(5): 547-553 (2001).

Westlind-Johnsson A, Malmebo S, Johansson A, et. al. Comparative analysis of 3A4 expression in human liver suggests only a minor role for CYP3A5 in drug metabolism. *Drug Metab Dispos.* 31(6):755-61 (2003).

Whirl-Carrillo M, McDonagh EM, Hebert JM, Gong L, Sangkuhl K, Thorn CF, et al. Pharmacogenomics knowledge for personalized medicine. *Clin Pharmacol Ther* 2012;92:414–7.

Wilkinson GR. Drug Metabolism and Variability among Patients in Drug Response. *NEJM* 2005; 352(21): 2211-21.

Winner J, Allen JD, Altar CA, Spahic-Mihajlovic A. Psychiatric pharmacogenomics predicts health resource utilization of outpatients with anxiety and depression. *Translational psychiatry.* 3:e242 (March 2013).

Wong SH, Happy C, Blinka D, Gock S, Jentzen JM, Donald Hon J, Coleman H, Jortani SA, Lucire Y, Morris-Kukoski CL, Neuman MG, Orsulak PJ, Sander T, Wagner MA, Wynn JR, Wu AH, Yeo KT. From personalized medicine to personalized justice: the promises of translational pharmacogenomics in the justice system. *Pharmacogenomics.* 2010 Jun;11(6):731-7..

Wrighton, S.A., VandenBranden, M. and Ring, B.J. The human drug metabolizing cytochromes P450. *Journal of Pharmacokinetics and Biopharmaceutics*. 24 (1996): 461–473.

Xie HG, Kim RB, Stein CM, Wilkinson GR, Wood AJJ. Genetic oplymorphism of (S)-mephenytoin 4'-hydroxylation in populations of African descent. *Br J Clin Pharmacol.* 1999;48:402-408.

Xie HG, Kim RB, Wood AJ, Stein CM. Molecular basis of ethnic differences in drug disposition and response *Annu Rev Pharmacol Toxicol.* 2001;41:815-50.

Yamaori S, Yamazaki H, Iwano S, et.al. Ethnic differences between Japanese and Caucasians in the expression levels of mRNAs for CYP3A4, CYP3A5 and CYP3A7: lack of co-regulation of the expression of CYP3A in Japanese livers. *Xenobiotica.* 35(1):69-83 (January 2005).

Zanger UM, Schwab M. Cytochrome P450 enzymes in drug metabolism: regulation of gene expression, enzyme activities, and impact of genetic variation. *Pharmacology & therapeutics.* 2013;138(1):103-41.

Zhang G, Zhang Y, Ling Y, Jia J. Web Resources for Pharmacogenomics. *Genomics Proteomics Bioinformatics* 13 (2015) 51–54.

Zhou SF, Di YM, Chan E, et al. Clinical pharmacogenetics and potential application in personalized medicine. *Curr Drug Metab.* 9:738–784 (2008).

Zhu B, Liu ZQ, Chen GL, Chen XP, Ou-Yang DS, Wang LS, et al. The distribution and gender difference of CYP3A activity in Chinese subjects. *Br J Clin Pharmacol.* 2003;55(3):264-9.

Historical Landmarks Leading to the Discovery of Pharmacogenetics

1866 Gregor Mendel established rules of heredity

1875 Francis Galton describes the concept of comparing pairs of monozygotic and dizygotic twins to distinguish genetic and environmental factors

1900–1913 William Bateson popularizes Mendelian inheritance, discovers linkage and introduces the term 'genetics'

1902–1909 Archibald Garrod develops the concept of "chemical individuality"

1932 Snyder established the monogenic inheritance of taste blindness for phenylthiocarbamide and documents "racial" differences in its incidence

1953 Bonicke, Reif and Hughes describe slow and rapid acetylation of isoniazide

1957 Kalow and Staron characterize serum cholinesterase deficiency in a subject with succinylcholine apnea

1957 Motulsky conceptualizes that inheritance might explain many individual differences in the efficacy and toxicity of drugs

1957–1970 Twin studies indicate polygenic influences on the pharmacogenetics of numerous drugs

1959 Vogel coins the term "pharmacogenetics"

1960 Evans establishes the genetic controls of isoniazide acetylation

1962 Kalow publishes the first monograph on pharmacogenetics: *Pharmacogenetics – the Heredity and the Response to Drugs*

1967–1973 Sjoqvist and his co-workers establish the metabolism of tricylic antidepressants is under genetic control

1975–1979 Smith (London) and Eichelbaum (Bonn) and their co-workers independently discover the debriscoquine/sparteine polymorphism of drug oxidation

1980 Discovery of the genetic polymorphism of thiopurine-methyltransferase (TPMT) by Weinshilboum and Sladek

1984 Description of the polymorphism of mephenytoin hydroxylation by Kupfer and Wedlund

1985 PCR allows genetic sequences to be amplified exponentially, accelerating Pharmacogenetics research

1988–1990 Gonzalez and Meyer collaborate to clone CYP2D6 and characterize the genetic defect of the debrisoquine/sparteine polymorphism

1990 Heim and Meyer publish the first allele-specific pharmacogenetic gene test for CYP2D6

1991 The first issue of the journal Pharmacogenetics is published

1993 Johansson, Ingelman-Sundberg and Bertilsson discover that stable gene amplifications of CYP2D6 cause the ultra-rapid-metabolizer phenotype

1994 Cloning and characterization of CYP2C19, which causes the mephenytoin polymorphism, by Goldstein et. al.

1995 A committee (Vatsis et.al.) offers nomenclature for NAT alleles

1995 Krynetzki et. al. publish the first mutations of the TPMT gene, from which a DNA test is derived

1999 A nomenclature website for the human cytochrome P450 (CYP) allele is established by an international committee

1999 A public/private collaboration, the 'SNP Consortium' provides public information on genomic diversity

2001 A draft of the human genome sequence is published

2003 The FDA issues draft guidelines for submission of pharmacogenetic data with new drug applications

2003 Start of the "HapMap" project for building a map of haplotype blocks

2003 The human genome sequence is (almost) completed

2004 Characterization of > 1.8 million SNPs by the SNP Consortium

This Table below lists the resources to obtain allele frequency information.'

Name	License	Comments
HapMap project	Free access	HapMap project focus on the characterization of common SNPs with a minor allele frequency (MAF) of $\geq 5\%$
1000 Genomes project	Free access	Based on the Extended HapMap Collection. 1000 Genome project captured up to 98% of the SNPs with a MAF of $\geq 1\%$ in 1092 individuals from 14 populations
The NHLBI Exome Sequencing Project	Free access	Project directed to discover genes responsible for heart, lung and blood disorder, decided to release the allele frequency of each variant detected in their exome sequencing project
The Personal Genome Project	Free access	Project has the genomes of 174 individuals and the exomes of over 400 volunteers available for download
NextCode Health	Commercial	40 million validated variants collected from the genotype of 140,000 volunteers from Iceland
CHARGE consortia	Fee for access and require permission from CHARGE consortia	1000 whole exome data sets of well-phenotyped individuals from the CHARGE consortium

ADDENDUM: POPULATION, DISEASE-SPECIFIC, AND SEQUENCE DATABASES

Population databases	
Exome Aggregation Consortium http://exac.broadinstitute.org/	Database of variants found during exome sequencing of 61,486 unrelated individuals sequenced as part of disease-specific and population genetic studies.
Exome Variant Server http://evs.gs.washington.edu/EVS	Database of variants found during exome sequencing of several large cohorts of European & African American ancestry individuals.
1000 Genomes Project http://browser.1000genomes.org	Database of variants found during low and high-coverage genomic and targeted sequencing from 26 populations. Provides more diversity compared to the EVS.
dbSNP http://www.ncbi.nlm.nih.gov/snp	Database of short genetic variations (≤50 bp) submitted from many sources. May lack details of the originating study and may contain pathogenic variants.
dbVar http://www.ncbi.nlm.nih.gov/dbvar	Database of structural variation (>50 bp) submitted from many sources.

Disease-specific databases

ClinVar http://www.ncbi.nlm.nih.gov/clinvar	Database of assertions about clinical significance and phenotype relationship of human variations.
OMIM http://www.omim.org	Database of human genes and genetic conditions that also contains representative sampling of disease-associated genetic variants.
Human Gene Mutation Database http://www.hgmd.org	Database of variant annotations published in literature.
Human Genome Variation Society http://www.hgvs.org/dblist/dblist.html Leiden Open Variation Database http://www.lovd.nl	HGVS site developed a list of thousands of databases that provide variant annotations on specific subsets of human variation. A large percentage of databases are built in the LOVD.
DECIPHER http://decipher.sanger.ac.uk	Molecular cytogenetic database for clinicians and researchers linking genomic microarray data with phenotype using the Ensembl genome browser.

Sequence databases

NCBI Genome http://www.ncbi.nlm.nih.gov/genome	Source of full human genome reference sequences
RefSeqGene http://www.ncbi.nlm.nih.gov/refseq/rsg	Medically relevant gene reference sequence resource.
Locus Reference Genomic http://www.lrg-sequence.org	
MitoMap http://www.mitomap.org/MITOMAP/	Revised Cambridge reference sequence for human mitochondrial DNA.

END NOTES

1.   Watson JD, Crick FH. Molecular structure of nucleic acids; a structure for deoxyribose nucleic acid. *Nature* 171 (4356): 737–738. (April 1953)

2.   Nebert, D. Zhang, G, Vesell ES. From Human Genetics and Genomics to Pharmacogenetics and Pharmacogenomics: past lessons, future directions. *Drug Metab. Rev.* 2008; 40(2): 187-224.

3.   Ibid, p. 188.

4.   Motulsky AG. Drug reactions enzymes, and biochemical genetics. *J Am Med Assoc.*1957;165:835–837

5.   Dreifus, C. A conversation with Arno Motulsky: A Genetics Pioneer Sees a Bright Future, Cautiously. *The New York Times.* April 29, 2008. [http://www.nytimes.com/2008/04/29/science]

6.   Vogel F. Moderne probleme der humangenetik. *Ergeb Inn Med Kinderheilkd.* 1959;12:52–125.

7.   Nebert, D. Zhang, G, Vesell ES. From Human Genetics and Genomics to Pharmacogenetics and Pharmacogenomics: past lessons, future directions. *Drug Metab. Rev.* 2008; 40(2): 187-224.

8.   Kalow, W. Pharmacogenetics – the Heredity and the Response to Drugs. *Journ. Pharmaceu. Sc.* Vol. 52. Issue 2. Feb 1963. P. 208.

9.   Sjöqvist, F. Hammer, W. et. Al. Plasma level of monomethylated tricyclic antidepressants and side effects in man. *Excepta Medica.* International Congress Series. No 145; p 246-257.

10. Vesell ES, Page JG. Genetic control of drug levels in man: phenylbutazone. *Science.* 1968;159:1479–1480.

11. K.F. Mullis, F. Faloona, S. Scharf, R. Saiki, G. Horn and H. Erlich, 1986, *Specific enzymatic amplification of DNA in vitro: the polymerase chain reaction.* Cold Spring Harbor Symposium in Quantitative Biology, 51:263–273.

12. Pharmacokinetics is, most simply, defined as what the body does to a drug. In contrast, pharmacodynamics is defined, most simply, as what the drug does to the body.

13. Schadt, E. Molecular Networks as Sensors and Drivers of Common Human Diseases. 461 *Nature* 218 (2001).

14. Ahmad A, Mast MR, Nijpels G, Elders PJ, Dekker JM, Hugtenburg JG. Identification of drug-related problems of elderly patients discharged from hospital. *Patient Prefer Adherence.* 2014;8:155-65.

15. Tulner LR, Frankfort SV, Gijsen GJ, van Campen JP, Koks CH, Beijnen JH. Drug-drug interactions in a geriatric outpatient cohort: prevalence and relevance. *Drugs Aging.* 2008;25(4):343-55.

16. Hohl CM, Dankoff J, Colacone A, Afilalo M. Polypharmacy, adverse drug-related events, and potential adverse drug interactions in elderly patients presenting to an emergency department. *Ann Emerg Med.* 2001;38(6):666-71.

17. Doucet J, Chassagne P, Trivalle C, Landrin I, Pauty MD, Kadri N, et al. Drug-drug interactions related to hospital admissions in older adults - a prospective study of 1000 patients. *American Geriatrics Society.* 1996;44(8).

18. Lindley CM, Tully MP, Paramsothy V, Tallis RC. Inappropriate Medication is a Major Cause of Adverse Drug Reactions in Elderly Patients. *Age Ageing.* 1992;21:294-300.

19. Beijer HJ, de Blaey CJ. Hospitalizations caused by adverse drug reactions (ADR): a meta-analysis of observational studies. *Pharm World Sci.* 2002 Apr;24(2):46-54.

20. Verbeurgt P, Mamiya T, Oesterheld J. How common are drug and gene interactions? Prevalence in a sample of 1143 patients with CYP2C9, CYP2C19 and CYP2D6 genotyping. *Pharmacogenomics* (2014) 15(5), 655–665.

21. Wilkinson GR. Drug Metabolism and Variability among Patients in Drug Response. *NEJM* 2005; 352(21): 2211-21.

22. Personalized Medicine Coalition. *The Case for Personalized Medicine*. 4th Edition 2014.

23. Goodall, D.S. The Molecular Perspective: Cytochrome P450. *The Oncologist.* April 2001 vol. 6 no. 2; p 205-206.

24. Verbeurgt P, Mamiya T, Oesterheld J. How common are drug and gene interactions? Prevalence in a sample of 1143 patients with CYP2C9, CYP2C19 and CYP2D6 genotyping. *Pharmacogenomics* (2014) 15(5), 655–665.

25. de Montello, ed. *Cytochrome P450 Structure, Mechanism and Biochemitry*, 3rd Ed. Kluwer Academic/Plenum Publishers. (2005).

26. Paine MF, Hart HL, Ludington SS, Haining RL, Rettie AE, Zeldin DC. The human intestinal cytochrome P450 "pie". *Drug Metab Dispos.* 2006 May;34(5):880-6.

27. Shimada T, Yamazaki H, Mimura M, Inui Y, Guengerich FP. Interindividual variations in human liver cytochrome P-450 enzymes involved in the oxidation of drugs, carcinogens and toxic chemicals: studies with liver microsomes of 30 Japanese and 30 Caucasians. *J Pharmacol Exp Ther.* 1994 Jul;270(1):414-23.

28. Preissner SC, Hoffmann MF, Preissner R, Dunkel M, Gewiess A and Preissner S. Polymorphic Cytochrome P450 Enzymes (CYPs) and Their Role in Personalized Therapy. *PLoS One.* 2013; 8(12): e82562.

29. Ibid, p. 17.

30. Mrazek, D. *Psychiatric Pharmacogenomics*. Oxford Un. Press, 2011. p3-6. 2010.

31. Data obtained in clinical practice of D. Durham, Genelex Corp. and Rennaissance Rx Corp.

32. Wong SH, Happy C, Blinka D, Gock S, Jentzen JM, Donald Hon J, Coleman H, Jortani SA, Lucire Y, Morris-Kukoski CL, Neuman MG, Orsulak PJ, Sander T, Wagner MA, Wynn JR, Wu AH, Yeo KT. From personalized medicine to personalized justice: the promises of translational pharmacogenomics in the justice system. *Pharmacogenomics.* 2010 Jun;11(6):731-7.

33. Sallee FR, DeVane CL, Ferrell RE: Fluoxetine-related death in a child with cytochrome P-450 2D6 genetic deficiency. *J. Child. Adolesc. Psychopharmacol.* 10, 327–334 (2000).

34. Leeder JS, Developmental Aspects of Drug Metabolism in Children. *Therapeutic Innovation & Regulatory Science* Oct 1996 vol. 30 no. 4 1135-1143.

35. Leeder JS, Kearns GL.Pharmacogenetics in pediatrics. Implications for practice. *Pediatr Clin North Am.* 1997 Feb;44(1):55-77.

36. Kearns GL, Leeder JS, Gaedigk A.Impact of the CYP2C19*17 allele on the pharmacokinetics of omeprazole and pantoprazole in children: evidence for a differential effect. *Drug Metab Dispos.* 2010 Jun;38(6):894-7.

37. Center for Devices and Radiologic Health, et.al. US Food and Drug Administration, Guidance for Industry and FDA Staff: Pharmacogenetic Tests and Geneitc Tests for Heritable Markers 3, (2007).

38. Restatement of Torts: Products Liability 6(c). (1998).

39. Redick, T P. Twenty-First Century Toxicogenomics Meets Twentieth Mass Tort Precedent: Is There a Duty to Warn of a "Hypothetical" Harm to an Eggshell Gene? 42 *Washburn Law J.* 547, 667 (2003).

40. Hamburg MA, Collins FS. The path to personalized medicine. *N Engl J Med.* 2010; 363(4):301-4.

41. *Larkin v. Pfizer, Inc.*, 152 S.W.3d 758, 763-64 (Ky. 2004).

42. *Perez v. Wyeth Labs, Inc.*, 734 A.2d 1245, 1255-56 (N.J. 1999).

43. *State ex rel.* Johnson & Johnson v. Karl, 647 S.E.2d 899, 910 (2007).

44. Healy D, Herxheimer A, Menkes DB: Antidepressants and violence: problems at the interface of medicine and law. *PloS* 3, 1478–1487 (2006).

45. Lucire Y, Crotty C. Antidepressant-induced akathisia-related homicides associated with diminishing mutations in metabolizing genes of the CYP450 family. *Pharmgenomics Pers Med.* 2011;4:65-81.

46. Healy, M. Doctors Untrained to Utilize Genetic Testing. *Los Angeles Times.* Oct 24, 2009. A19.

47. *Thinking Outside the Pillbox A System-wide Approach to Improving Patient Medication Adherence for Chronic Disease.* A NEHI Research Brief. August 2009.

48. Classen DC, Pestotnik SL, Evans RS, et al. Adverse drug events in hospitalized patients. *JAMA* 1997;277(4):301-6.

49. Cullen DJ, Bates DW, Small SD, et al. The incident reporting system does not detect adverse drug events: A problem for quality improvement. *Journal on Quality Improvement* 1995;21(10):541-8.

50. Ibid and Lazarou J, Pomeranz BH, Corey PN. Incidence of adverse drug reactions in hospitalized patients: a meta-analysis of prospective studies. *JAMA.* 1998;279(15): 1200-1205.

51. Tulner LR, Frankfort SV, et.al. Drug-drug interactions in a geriatric outpatient cohort: prevalence and relevance. *Drugs Aging.* 2008; 25(4):343-355.

52. http://www.ncbi.nlm.nih.gov/gtr/

53. Relling, MV, Klein, TE. CPIC: Clinical Pharmacogenetics Implementation Consortium of the Pharmacogenomics Research Network. *Clinical Pharmacology and Therapeutics.* Vol.89. No.3. March (2011).

54. Mrazek, D. *Psychiatric Pharmacogenomics.* Oxford Un. Press, 2011.

55. Eugenics: a science that tries to improve the human race by controlling which people become parents. Merriam-Webster Dictionary: http://www.merriam-webster.com/dictionary/eugenics.

56. Personalized Medicine Coalition. *The Case for Personalized Medicine.* 4th Edition 2014.

57. Definition of "underwriting" includes rules for, or determination of, benefits eligibility, the computation of premium or contribution amounts, the application of any preexisting condition exclusion and, other activities related to the creation, renewal or replacement of a health insurance contract. GINA Title I, § 101(d) (amending ERISA, 29U.S.C. 1191b(d)(9); GINA Title I, § 102(a)(4) (amending the PHS Act with respect to group markets, 42 U.S.C. 300gg-91(d)(19)); GINA Title I, § 103(d) (amending IRS Code, 26 U.S.C. 9832(d)(10)); GINA Title I, § 104(b)(1)(amending the Social Security Act with respect to medigap, 42 U.S.C. 1395ss(x)(3)(E)); GINA Title I, § 105(a) amending HIPAA, 42 U.S.C. 1320d-9(b)(1)).

58. GINA Title I, § 101(a)(2) (amending ERISA, 29 U.S.C. 1182(b)(3)(A)); GINA Title I, § 102(a)(1) (amending the PHS Act with respect to group markets, 42 U.S.C. 300gg-1(b)(3)(A)) (prohibiting group-based discrimination by group health plans). GINA Title I, § 101(b) (amending ERISA, 29 U.S.C. 1182(d)(1), (2)); GINA Title I, § 102(a)(2) (amending the PHS Act with respect to group markets, 42 U.S.C. 300gg-1(d)(1), (2)); GINA Title I, § 103(b) (amending IRS Code, 26 U.S.C. 9802(d)(1), (2)); GINA Title I, § 104(b)(1) (amending Social Security Act with respect to medigap, 42 U.S.C. 4395(ss)(x)(2)(A), (B)) (prohibiting use of genetic information by group plans for underwriting purposes and prior to enrollment). GINA Title I, § 103(a)(2) (amending IRS Code, 26 U.S.C. 9802(b)(3)(A)) (prohibiting the use of genetic information by group plans in determining premium and contribution amounts). GINA Title I, § 102(b)(1) (amending the PHS

Act with respect to individual markets, 42 U.S.C. 300gg-53(a)(1), (b)(1), (c)(1), (e)(1), (2))
(prohibiting use of genetic information by insurers in the individual market in making
determinations for eligibility, coverage, preexisting conditions, premium and contribution rates, for
underwriting purposes and prior to enrollment). GINA Title I, § 104(a) (amending Social Security
Act with respect to medigap, 42 U.S.C. 1395ss(s)(2)(E)) (prohibiting use of genetic information by
Medicare Supplemental Policies in making determinations for eligibility, coverage, preexisting
condition, premium or contribution rates).

59. Department of Labor website, "FAQs on the Genetic Nondiscrimination Information Act",
     Question 7 (available at www.dol.gov/ebsa/faqs/faq-GINA.html).

60. GINA Title I, § 101(b) (amending ERISA, 29 U.S.C. 1182(c)(1), (d)(1), (2)); GINA Title I, §
     102(a)(2) (amending the PHS Act with respect to group markets, 42 U.S.C. 300gg-1(c)(1), (d)(1),
     (2)); GINA Title I, § 102(b)(1) (amending the PHS Act with respect to individual markets, 42
     U.S.C. 300gg-53(d)(1), (e)(1), (2)); GINA Title I, § 103(b) (amending IRS Code, 26 U.S.C.
     9802(c)(1), (d)(1), (2)); GINA Title I, § 104(b)(1) (amending the Social Security Act with respect
     to medigap, 42 U.S.C. 1395ss(x)(1)(A), (2)(A), (B)).

61. GINA Title I, § 101(b) (amending ERISA, 29 U.S.C. 1182(c)(3)); GINA Title I, § 102(a)(2)
     (amending the PHS Act with respect to group markets, 42 U.S.C. 300gg-1(c)(3)); GINA Title I, §
     102(b)(1) (amending the PHS Act with respect to individual markets, 42 U.S.C. 300gg-53(d)(3));
     GINA Title I, § 103(b) (amending IRS Code, 26 U.S.C. 9802(c)(3)); GINA Title I, § 104(b)(1)
     (amending the Social Security Act with respect to medigap, 42 U.S.C. 1395ss(s)(2)(F)).

62. GINA Title I, § 101(b) (amending ERISA, 29 U.S.C. 1182(c)(4)); GINA Title I, § 102(a)(2)
     (amending the PHS Act with respect to group markets, 42 U.S.C. 300gg-1(c)(3)); GINA Title I, §
     102(b)(1) (amending the PHS Act with respect to individual markets, 42 U.S.C. 300gg-53(d)(4));
     GINA Title I, § 103(b) (amending IRS Code, 26 U.S.C. 9802(c)(4)); GINA Title I, § 104(b)(1)
     (amending the Social Security Act with respect to medigap, 42 U.S.C. 1395ss(x)(1)(D)).

63. GINA Title I, § 101(b) (amending ERISA, 29 U.S.C. 1182(d)(3)); GINA Title I, § 102(a)(2)
     (amending the PHS Act with respect to group markets, 42 U.S.C. 300gg-1(d)(3)); GINA Title I, §
     102(b)(1) (amending the PHS Act with respect to individual markets, 42 U.S.C. 300gg-53(e)(3));
     GINA Title I, § 103(b) (amending IRS Code, 26 U.S.C. 9802(d)(3)); GINA Title I, § 104(b)(1)
     (amending the Social Security Act with respect to medigap, 42 U.S.C. 1395ss(x)(2)(C)).

64. Paulozzi, L. Div of Unintentional Injury Prevention; Annest J. Office of Statistics and
     Programming, National Center for Injury Prevention and Control. United States Centers for
     Disease Control. *Unintentional Poisoning Deaths – United States 1999- 2004*. (2005).

65. http://www.cdc.gov/homeandrecreationalsafety/overdose/facts.html

66. Substance Abuse and Mental Health Services Administration. Highlights of the 2011 Drug Abuse
     Warning Network (DAWN) findings on drug-related emergency department visits. The DAWN
     Report. Rockville, MD: US Department of Health and Human Services, Substance Abuse and
     Mental Health Services Administration; 2013. Available from
     URL: http://www.samhsa.gov/data/2k13/DAWN127/sr127-DAWN-highlights.htm

67. Berenbeim DM. Polypharmacy: overdosing on good intentions. *Manag Care Q.* 2002;10(3):1-5.

68. Preskorn SH, Kane CP, Lobello K, et al. Cytochrome P450 2D6 phenoconversion is common in
     patients being treated for depression: implications for personalized medicine. *J Clin Psychiatry.*
     2013;74(6):614-621.

69. Hohl CM, Dankoff J, Colacone A, Afilalo M. Polypharmacy, adverse drug-related events, and
     potential adverse drug interactions in elderly patients presenting to an emergency department. *Ann
     Emerg Med.* 2001;38(6):666-671.

70. http://youscript.com/healthcare-professionals/what-is-youscript/

71. Durham, D. Utilizing Pharmacogenetic Testing in Psychiatry – data from the New Mexico
     cohort. http://www.healthshire.com/utilizing-pharmacogenetic-testing-in-psychiatry-the-time-is-
     now%e2%80%a8/

72. Runde I, et. al., 2011, *Translational Psychiatry.*

73. Mrazek, D. *Clinical Implementation of Psychiatric Pharmacogenomic Testing: characterizing and displaying genetic variants for clinical action.* Mayo Clinic. December 2, 2011.

74. Hall-Flavin DK, Winner JG, Allen JD, Jordan JJ, Nesheim RS, Snyder KA, et al. Using a pharmacogenomic algorithm to guide the treatment of depression. *Transl Psychiatry.* 2012;2:e172.

75. Winner, J, Allen JD, et.al. Psychiatric pharmacogenomics predicts health resource utilizaton of outpatients with anxiety and depression. *Transl Psychiatry.* March: 3(3). 2013. Published online March 19, 2013.

76. Chou, WH, Yan FX, et.al. Extension of a pilot study: impact from the cytochrome P450 2D6 polymorphism on outcome and costs associated with severe mental illness. *J Clin Psychopharmacol.* 2000 April; 20(2):246-51.

77. Ruano G, Szarek B, Villagra D, Gorowski K, et al. Length of psychiatric hospitalization is correlated with CYP2D6 functional status in inpatients with major despressive disorder. *Biomarkers Med.* 7(3), 429-439 (2013)..

78. Alagoz O, Durham D, Kasirajan K. (2015) Cost Effectiveness of One-Time Genetic Testing to Minimize Lifetime Adverse Drug Reactions. *The Pharmacogenomics Journal.* 19 May 2015 Issue. 39:1-8.

79. Winner J, Allen JD, Altar CA, Spahic-Mihajlovic A. Psychiatric pharmacogenomics predicts health resource utilization of outpatients with anxiety and depression. *Translational psychiatry.* 2013;3:e242.

80. Hall-Flavin DK, Winner JG, Allen JD, Carhart JM, Proctor B, Snyder KA, et al. Utility of integrated pharmacogenomic testing to support the treatment of major depressive disorder in a psychiatric outpatient setting. *Pharmacogenetics and genomics* 2013;23(10):535-48.

81. Biskupiak J, Biltaji E, Bress A, Ye X, Unni S, Newman R, Ashcraft A, Mamiya T, Brixner D. Cost-consequence analysis for pharmacogenetic testing in an Elderly Population. Journal of Managed Care & Specialty Pharmacy. Oct 2015. Vol.21, No. 10-a: S81.

82. Brixner D, Biltaji E, Bress A, Unni S, Ye X, Mamiya T, Ashcraft A, Biskupiak J. The effect of pharmacogenetic profiling with a clinical decision support tool on healthcare resource utilization and estimated costs in the elderly exposed to polypharmacy. Journal of Medical Economics. 2016;19(3):213-28.

83. Biskupiak J, Unni S, Thirumaran RK, Biltaji E, Bress A, Ye X, Ashcraft K, Brixner D. Impact of pharmacogenetics with integrated clinical decision support on healthcare utilization and costs in the elderly receiving polypharmacy: Report update. 2016. (Unpublished Data)

84. Recall that CYP2D6 is a high affinity and low capacity enzyme and CYP3A4 is a high capacity and low affinity enzyme.

85. Villagra, D. *et al.* Novel drug metabolism indices for pharmacogenetic functional status based on combinatory genotyping of CYP2C9, CYP2C19 and CYP2D6 genes. *Biomarkers in medicine* 5, 427-438 (2011).

86. Hocum B, White JR, Heck J, Thirumaran RK, Moyer N, Newman R & Ashcraft K. Cytochrome P450 gene testing & drug interaction analysis in mixed-race, U.S. patients referred for Pharmacogenetic testing. *American Journal of Health-System Pharmacy* 2016 Jan 15; 73(2):61-7.

87. Ingelman-Sundberg M. Genetic polymorphisms of cytochrome P450 2D6 (CYP2D6): clinical consequences, evolutionary aspects and functional diversity. Karolinska Institute. *The Pharmacogenomics Journal.* 5, 6–13. doi:10.1038/sj.tpj.6500285. October (2004).

88. Recent data has shown that Pacific Islanders have a high frequency of reduced functioning CYP2D610*10 allele. Thus, it is currently estimated that about 30 percent of this population are intermediate metabolizers. Additionally there are frequencies of functional and non-functional allele frequencies that differ substantially between African-Americans and Africans. Only African-

Americans will be addressed herein as the data for East African populations are still highly approximated.

89. Mrazek, D. *Psychiatric Pharmacogenomics*. Oxford Un. Press, 2011. P48-49.

90. , Groen DK, Phelps MA, Sadee W. Pharmacogenomic testing: relevance in medical practice: why drugs work in some patients but not in others. *Cleve Clin J Med*. 2011 Apr;78(4):243-57

91. Ma Q, Lu AY. Pharmacogenetics, pharmacogenomics, and individualized medicine. *Pharmacol Rev.* 2011 Jun;63(2):437-59.

92. Ibid.

93. Kirchheiner J, Nickchen K, Bauer M, et al. Pharmacogenetics of antidepressants and antipsychotics: the contribution of allelic variations to the phenotype of drug response. *Mol Psychiatry*. 2004;9:442–473.

94. Robert, J., Le Morvan, V., Giovannetti, E., Peters, G.J. & EORTC, P.G.o. On the use of pharmacogenetics in cancer treatment and clinical trials. *European journal of cancer* 50, 2532-43 (2014).

95. Robarge, J.D., Li, L., Desta, Z., Nguyen, A. & Flockhart, D.A. The star-allele nomenclature: retooling for translational genomics. *Clinical pharmacology and therapeutics* 82, 244-8 (2007).

96. Hein, D.W., Boukouvala, S., Grant, D.M., Minchin, R.F. & Sim, E. Changes in consensus arylamine N-acetyltransferase gene nomenclature. *Pharmacogenetics and genomics* 18, 367-8 (2008).

97. Robarge, J.D., Li, L., Desta, Z., Nguyen, A. & Flockhart, D.A. The star-allele nomenclature: retooling for translational genomics. *Clinical pharmacology and therapeutics* 82, 244-8 (2007).

98. http://www.cypalleles.ki.se/.

99. http://bioinformatics.charite.de/supercyp/

100. Kalman LV., et.al Pharmacogenetic allele nomenclature: International workgroup recommendations for test result reporting. *Clinical Pharmacology & Therapeutics 2016 Feb; 99(2):172-85.*

101. Crews KR, Gaedigk A, Dunnenberger HM, Leeder JS *et al*. Clinical Pharmacogenetics Implementation Consortium guidelines for cytochrome P450 2D6 genotype and codeine therapy: 2014 update *Clin Pharmacol Ther*. 2014 Apr;95(4):376-82.

102. de Leon J, Susce MT, Johnson M, Hardin M, Maw L, Shao A et al. DNA Microarray Technology in the Clinical Environment: The AmpliChip CYP450 Test for CYP2D6 and CYP2C19 Genotyping. *CNS Spectr*. 2009;14(1):19-34.

103. Lyon E, Foster JG, Palomaki GE, Pratt VM, Reynolds K, Sabato MF et al. Laboratory testing of CYP2D6 alleles in relation to tamoxifen therapy. *Genet Med*. 2012;14(12):990-1000.

104. Man M, Farmen M, Dumaual C, Teng CH, Moser B, Irie S *et al*. Genetic variation in metabolizing enzyme and transporter genes: comprehensive assessment in 3 major East Asian subpopulations with comparison to Caucasians and Africans. *J Clin Pharmacol*. 2010 Aug;50(8):929-40.

105. Kiyotani K, Shimizu M, Kumai T, Kamataki T, Kobayashi S, Yamazaki H. Limited effects of frequent CYP2D6*36-*10 tandem duplication allele on in vivo dextromethorphan metabolism in a Japanese population. *Eur J Clin Pharmacol*. 2010 Oct;66(10):1065-8.

106. Cai WM, Nikoloff DM, Pan RM, de Leon J, Fanti P, Fairchild M *et al*. CYP2D6 genetic variation in healthy adults and psychiatric African-American subjects: implications for clinical practice and genetic testing. *Pharmacogenomics J*. 2006 Sep-Oct;6(5):343-50.

107. Hocum B, White JR, Heck J, Thirumaran RK, Moyer N, Newman R & Ashcraft K. Cytochrome P450 gene testing & drug interaction analysis in mixed-race, U.S. patients referred for Pharmacogenetic testing. *American Journal of Health-System Pharmacy* 2016 Jan 15; 73(2):61-7.

108. http://www.fda.gov/Drugs/ScienceResearch/ResearchAreas/Pharmacogenetics/ucm083378.htm..

109. Desta Z, Zhao X, Shin JG, Flockhart DA. Clinical significance of the cytochrome P450 2C19 genetic polymorphism. *Clin Pharmacokinet.* 2002;41(12):913-58.

110. Mrazek, D. *Psychiatric Pharmacogenomics.* Oxford Un. Press, 2011. (2010).

111. Li-Wan-Po A., Girard T., et. al. Pharmacogenetics of CYP2C19: functional and clinical implications of a new variant CYP2C19*17. *Br J Clin Pharmacol.* 69(3): 222–230 (March 2010).

112. Mrazek, D. *Psychiatric Pharmacogenomics.* Oxford Un. Press, 2011. (2010).

113. Wang G, Lei HP, Li Z, Tan ZR, Guo D, Fan L, Chen Y, Hu DL, Wang D, Zhou HH. The CYP2C19 ultra-rapid metabolizer genotype influences the pharmacokinetics of voriconazole in healthy male volunteers. *Eur J Clin Pharmacol.*65:281–5 (2009).

114. Rosemary J, Adithan C. The Pharmacogenetics of CYP2C9 and CYP2C19: Ethnic Variation and Clinical Significance. *Current Clinical Pharmacology.* 2007;2:93-109.

115. Simon T, Verstuyft C, Mary-Krause M, Quteineh L, Drouet E, Méneveau N, et al. Genetic Determinants of Response to Clopidogrel and Cardiovascular Events. *NEJM.* 2009;360(4):363-75.

116. Li-Wan-Po A., Girard T., et. al. Pharmacogenetics of CYP2C19: functional and clinical implications of a new variant CYP2C19*17. *Br J Clin Pharmacol.* 2010 March; 69(3): 222–230.

117. Mejin M, Tiong WN, Lai LYH, Tiong LL, Bujang AM, Hwang SS et al. CYP2C19 genotypes and their impact on clopidogrel responsiveness in percuteneous coronary intervention. *Int J Clin Pharm.* 2013;35:621-28.

118. Phillips KA, Veenstra DL, Oren E, Lee JK, Sadee W. Potential Role of Pharmacogenomics in Reducing Adverse Drug Reactions: A Systematic Review. *JAMA.* 2001;286:2270-2279.

119. Xie HG, Kim RB, Stein CM, Wilkinson GR, Wood AJJ. Genetic oplymorphism of (S)-mephenytoin 4'-hydroxylation in populations of African descent. *Br J Clin Pharmacol.* 1999;48:402-408.

120. Sim SC, Risinger C, Dahl ML, Aklillu E, Christensen M, Bertilsson L et al. A common novel CYP2C19 gene variant causes ultrarapid drug metabolism relevant for the drug response to proton pump inhibitors and antidepressants. *Clin Pharmacol Ther.* 2006;79:103-13.

121. Xie HG, Kim RB, Wood AJ, Stein CM. Molecular basis of ethnic differences in drug disposition and response *Annu Rev Pharmacol Toxicol.* 2001;41:815-50.

122. Hocum B, White JR, Heck J, Thirumaran RK, Moyer N, Newman R & Ashcraft K. Cytochrome P450 gene testing & drug interaction analysis in mixed-race, U.S. patients referred for Pharmacogenetic testing. *American Journal of Health-System Pharmacy* 2016 Jan 15; 73(2):61-7.

123. Samer CF, Lorenzini KI, Rollason V, Daali Y, Desmeules JA. Applications of CYP450 testing in the clinical setting. *Molecular diagnosis & therapy.* 2013;17(3):165-84.

124. Rettie AE, Jones JP. Clinical and Toxicological Relevance of CYP2C9: Drug-Drug Interactions and Pharmacogenetics. *Annu. Rev. Pharmacol. Toxicol.* 2005;45:477-94.

125. Ingelman-Sundberg M. Genetic polymorphisms of cytochrome P450 2D6 (CYP2D6): clinical consequences, evolutionary aspects and functional diversity. Karolinska Institute. *The Pharmacogenomics Journal.* 5, 6–13 (October 2004).

126. Mrazek, D. *Psychiatric Pharmacogenomics.* Oxford Un. Press, (2011).

127. Scordo M, Aklillu E, et al. Genetic polymorphism of cytochrome P450 2C9 in a Caucasian and a black African population. Br *J Clin Pharmacol.* 2001 October; 52(4): 447–450.

128. Zhou SF, Liu JP, Chowbay B. Polymorphism of human cytochrome P450 enzymes and its clinical impact. *Drug Metabolism Reviews.* 2009; 41(2):89-295.

129. Van Booven D, Marsh S, McLeod H, Carrillo MW, Sangkuhl K, Klein TE, Altman RB: Cytochrome P450 2C9-CYP2C9. *Pharmacogenet Genomics*. 2010 Apr;20(4):277-81.

130. Horn, J, Hansten, D. Get to Know an Enzyme: CYP2C9. *Pharmacy Times*. March (2008) Publ http://www.pharmacytimes.com/publications/issue/2008/2008-03/2008-03-8462#sthash.iZ8anpjl.dpuf

131. Wen X, Wang JS, et al. In vitro evaluation of valproic acid as an inhibitor of human cytochrome P450 isoforms: preferential inhibition of cytochrome P450 2C9 (CYP2C9). *Britich J. Clin. Pharmacol.* Nov;52(5): 547-553 (2001).

132. Ho PC, Abbott FS, et al. Influence of CYP2C9 genotypes on the formation of a hepatotoxic metabolite of valproic acid in human liver microsomes. *Pharmacogenomic J.* 3(6):335-42 (2003).

133. Scott SA, Khasawneh R, Peter I, Kornreich R, Desnick RJ. Combined CYP2C9, VKORC1 and CYP4F2 frequencies among racial and ethnic groups. Pharmacogenomics. 2010;11(6):781-91.

134. http://www.fda.gov/Drugs/ScienceResearch/ResearchAreas/Pharmacogenetics/ucm083378

135. Hocum B, White JR, Heck J, Thirumaran RK, Moyer N, Newman R & Ashcraft K. Cytochrome P450 gene testing & drug interaction analysis in mixed-race, U.S. patients referred for Pharmacogenetic testing. *American Journal of Health-System Pharmacy* 2016 Jan 15; 73(2):61-7.

136. Thorn CF, Aklillu E, Klein TE, Altman RB. PharmGKB summary: very important pharmacogene information for CYP1A2. *Pharmacogenetics and genomics*. 2012;22(1):73-7

137. Perera V, Gross AS, Polasek TM, Qin Y, Rao G, Forrest A, et al. Considering CYP1A2 phenotype and genotype for optimizing the dose of olanzapine in the management of schizophrenia. *Expert opinion on drug metabolism & toxicology*. 2013;9(9):1115-37.

138. Bozina N, Bradamante V, Lovric M. Genetic polymorphism of metabolic enzymes P450 (CYP) as a susceptibility factor for drug response, toxicity, and cancer risk. *Arh Hig Rada Toksikol.* 2009;60(2):217-42.

139. Wrighton, S.A., VandenBranden, M. and Ring, B.J. The human drug metabolizing cytochromes P450. *Journal of Pharmacokineticsand Biopharmaceutics*. 24 (1996): 461–473.

140. Niwa, Toshiro, Murayama, Norie and Yamazaki, Hiroshi. Comparison of the Contributions of Cytochromes P450 3A4 and 3A5 in Drug Oxidation Rates and Substrate Inhibition. *Journal of Health Science*, 56(2010): 239-256.

141. Frye, R.F., Chapter 3: Pharmacogenetics of Oxidative Drug Metabolism and its clinical applications. *Pharmacogenomics: Applications to Patient Care*. (Washington, D.C: American College of Clinical Pharmacy, 2009).

142. Kapelyukh Y, Paine MJ, Marechal JD, Sutcliffe MJ, Wolf CR, Roberts GC. Multiple substrate binding by cytochrome P450 3A4: estimation of the number of bound substrate molecules. *Drug Metab Dispos.* 2008;36(10):2136-44.

143. Evans WE, Relling RV: Pharmacogenomics: translating functional genomics into rational therapeutics. *Science* 1999;486:487-491.

144. Lamda JK, Lin YS, Schuetz EG, Thummel KE: Genetic contribution to variable human CYP3A-mediated metabolism. *Adv Drug Deliv Rev* 2002;18:1271-1294

145. Zhu B, Liu ZQ, Chen GL, Chen XP, Ou-Yang DS, Wang LS, et al. The distribution and gender difference of CYP3A activity in Chinese subjects. *Br J Clin Pharmacol.* 2003;55(3):264-9.

146. Shimada T, Yamazaki H, Mimura M, Inui Y, Guengerich FP. Interindividual variations in human liver cytochrome P-450 enzymes involved in the oxidation of drugs, carcinogens and toxic chemicals: studies with liver microsomes of 30 Japanese and 30 Caucasians. *J Pharmacol Exp Ther.* 1994;270(1):414-23.

147. Zanger UM, Schwab M. Cytochrome P450 enzymes in drug metabolism: regulation of gene expression, enzyme activities, and impact of genetic variation. *Pharmacology & therapeutics.* 2013;138(1):103-41.

148. Wang D, Guo Y, Wrighton SA, et al: Intronic polymorphism in *CYP3A4* affects hepatic expression and response to statin drugs. *Pharmacogenomics* J 2011;11:274-286.

149. Elens L, van Gelder T, Hesselink DA, Haufroid V, van Schaik RH. CYP3A4*22: promising newly identified CYP3A4 variant allele for personalizing pharmacotherapy. *Pharmacogenomics.* 2013;14(1):47-62.

150. Birdwell KA, Decker B, Barbarino JM, et al. : Clinical pharmacogenetics implementation consortium (CPIC) guidelines for CYP3A5 genotype and tacrolimus dosing. *Clin Pharmacol Ther.* 2015 Jul;98(1):19-24.

151. Lamba JK, Lin YS, Schuetz EG, Thummel KE. Genetic contribution to variable human CYP3A-mediated metabolism. *Adv Drug Deliv Rev.* 2002 Nov 18; 54(10):1271-94

152. Ibid: 1271-94.

153. Daly AK. Significance of the minor cytochrome P450 3A isoforms. *Clin Pharmacokinet.* 2006;45(1):13-31.

154. Quaranta S, Chevalier D, Allorge D, Lo-Guidice JM, et. al. Ethnic differences in the distribution of CYP3A5 gene polymorphisms. *Xenobiotica.* 2006, 36(12):1191-1200.

155. Roy JN, Lajoie J, Zijenah LS, Barama A, et. al. CYP3A5 genetic polymorphisms in different ethnic populations. *Drug Metab Dispos.* 2005, **33**(7):884-887.

156. *Specifically, the CYP3A5*7* polymorphism is believed to hold the most clinical significance.

157. Van Schaik, R.H., van der Heiden, I.P., van den Anker, J.N. & Lindemans, J. CYP3A5 variant allele frequencies in Dutch Caucasians. *Clinical chemistry 2002;* 48, 1668-7.

158. He P, Court MH, Greenblatt DJ, Von Moltke LL. Genotype-phenotype associations of cytochrome P450 3A4 and 3A5 polymorphism clearance in vivo. *Clin Pharmacaol Ther.* 2005 May; 77(5): 373-87.

159. Floyd MD, Gervasini G, Masica Al, et. al. Genotyp-phenotyp associations for common CYP3A4 and CYP3A5 variants in the basal and induced metabolism of midazolam in European and African-American men and women. *Pharmacogenetics.* 2003 Oct; 13(10:595-606.

160. Westlind-Johnsson A, Malmebo S, Johansson A, et. al. Comparative analysis of 3A4 expression in human liver suggests only a minor role for CYP3A5 in drug metabolism. *Drug Metab Dispos.* 2003;31(6):755-61.

161. Ibid.

162. Yamaori S, Yamazaki H, Iwano S, et.al. Ethnic differences between Japanese and Caucasians in the expression levels of mRNAs for CYP3A4, CYP3A5 and CYP3A7: lack of co-regulation of the expression of CYP3A in Japanese livers. *Xenobiotica.* 2005 Jan;35(1):69-83.

163. Birdwell KA, Decker B, Barbarino JM, et al. : Clinical pharmacogenetics implementation consortium (CPIC) guidelines for CYP3A5 genotype and tacrolimus dosing. *Clin Pharmacol Ther.* 2015 Jul;98(1):19-24.

164. Provenzani A, Notarbartolo M, Labbozzetta M, Poma P, Vizzini G, Salis P *et al.*: Influence of CYP3A5 and ABCB1 gene polymorphisms and other factors on tacrolimus dosing in Caucasian liver and kidney transplant patients. *Int J Mol Med.* 2011 Dec;28(6):1093-102.

165. Verbeurgt P, Mamiya T, Oesterheld J. How common are drug and gene interactions? Prevalence in a sample of 1143 patients with CYP2C9, CYP2C19 and CYP2D6 genotyping. *Pharmacogenomics.* 2014;15(5):655-65.

166. Hocum B, White JR, Heck J, Thirumaran RK, Moyer N, Newman R & Ashcraft K. Cytochrome P450 gene testing & drug interaction analysis in mixed-race, U.S. patients referred for Pharmacogenetic testing. *American Journal of Health-System Pharmacy* 2016 Jan 15; 73(2):61-7.

167. Abilify has about a 2 to 3 day half-life.

168. Fluoxetine is almost universally covered and on almost all insurance drug formularies.

169. Ring BJ, Catlow J, Lindsay TJ, Gillespie T, Roskos LK, Cerimele BJ, et al. Identification of the human cytochromes P450 responsible for the in vitro formation of the major oxidative metabolites of the antipsychotic agent olanzapine. *J Pharmacol Exp Ther* 1996;276:658-66.

170. Lyon, ER. A review of the effects of nicotine on schizophrenia and antipsychotic medications. *Psychatr. Serv.* 1999. Oct:50(10): 1346-50.

171. Nicotine, however, is thought to be predominantly metabolized by the CYP2A6 enzyme, and has only secondary interactions with the CYP1A2 enzyme (via O-demethylation with CYP2E1 of the Nicotine analogue GTS-21)). Hukkanen, A. Jacob, P. Benowitz, N. Metabolism and Disposition Kinetics of Nicotine. *Pharmacological Reviews.* Vol. 57, No. 1; 79-115. March 2005.

172. Callaghan JT, Bergstrom RF, Ptak LR, Beasley CM. Olanzapine: pharmacokinetic and pharmacodynamic profile. *Clin Pharmacokinet.* 1999;37:177-93.

173. Mäenpää J, Wrighton S, Bergstrom R, Cerimele B, Tatum D, Hatcher B, et al. Pharmacokinetic and pharmacodynamic interactions between fluvoxamine and olanzapine. *Clin Pharmacol Ther.* 1997;61:225.

174. Lucas RA, Gilfillan DJ, Bergstrom RF. A pharmacokinetic interaction between carbamazepine and olanzapine: observations on possible mechanism. *Eur J Clin Pharmacol.* 1998;54:639-43.

175. Olesen OV, Linnet K. Olanzapine serum concentrations in psychiatric patients given standard doses: the influence of co-medication. *Ther Drug Metab.* 1999;21:87-90.

176. Kraupl TF: Loss of libido in depression. *BMJ.* 1:305, 1972.

177. Segraves RT: Effects of psychotropic drugs on human erection and ejaculation. *Arch Gen Psychiatry.* 46:275-284, 1989.

178. Ashton AK, Hamer R, Rosen R: Serotonin reuptake inhibitor-induced sexual dysfunction and its treatment: A large-scale retrospective study of 596 psychiatric outpatients. *J Sex Marital Ther.* 23(3):165-175, 1997.

179. Goldbloom DS, Kennedy SH: Adverse interaction of fluoxetine and cyproheptadine in two patients with bulimia nervosa. *J Clin Psychiatry.* 52:261-262, 1991.

180. Mc Cormick S, Olin J, Brotman AW: Reversal of fluoxetine-induced anorgasmia by cyproheptadine in two patients. *J Clin Psychiatry.* 51:383-384, 1990.

181. Katz RJ, Rosenthal M: Adverse interaction of cyproheptadine with serotonergic antidepressants. *J Clin Psychiatry.* 55:314-315, 1994.

182. Norden MJ. Buspirone treatment of sexual dysfunction associated with selective serotonin reuptake inhibitors. *Depression.* 2:109-112, 1994.

183. Reynolds RD: Sertraline-induced anorgasmia treated with intermittent nefazodone. *J Clin Psychiatry.* 58:89, 1997.

184. Timmer CJ, Sitsen JM, Delbressine LP. Clinical Pharmacokinetics of Mirtazepine. *Clinical Pharmacokinetics.* June; 38(6) 461-74, 2000.

185. Aizenberg D, Gur S, Zemishlany Z, et al: Mianserin, a 5-HT2a/2c and alpha 2 antagonist, in the treatment of sexual dysfunction induced by serotonin reuptake inhibitors. *Clin Neuropharmacol.* 20(3):210-214, 1997.

186. Balogh S, Hendricks SE, Kang J: Treatment of fluoxetine-induced anorgasmia with amantadine. *J Clin Psychiatry.* 53:212-213, 1992.

187. Shrivastava RK, Shrivastava S, Overweg N, et al: Amantadine in the treatment of sexual dysfunction associated with selective serotonin reuptake inhibitors. J Clin Psychopharmacol. 15:83-84, 1993.

188. Balon R: Intermittent amantadine for fluoxetine-induced anorgasmia. *J Sex Marital Ther.* 22: 290-292, 1996.

189. Morales A, Condra M, Owen JA, et al: Is yohimbine effective in the treatment of organic impotence? Results of a controlled trial. *J Urol.* 137:1168-1172, 1987.

190. Hollander E, McCarley A: Yohimbine treatment of sexual side effects induced by serotonin reuptake blockers. *J Clin Psychiatry.* 53(6):207-209, 1992.

191. Price J, Grunhaus LJ: Treatment of clomipramine-induced anorgasmia with yohimbine: A case report. *J Clin Psychiatry.* 51:32-33, 1990.

192. Jacobsen FM: Fluoxetine-induced sexual dysfunction and an open trial of yohimbine. *J Clin Psychiatry.* 53:119-122, 1992.

193. Cohen AJ: Gingko biloba for drug-induced sexual dysfunction. Abstracts of the Annual Meeting of the American Psychiatric Association, San Diego, Calif., 1997, p 15.

194. Higgins, A. Nash, M. Lynch, A. Antidepressant-associated sexual dysfunction: impact, effects, and treatment. *Drug Health & Patient Safety.* 2010; 2: 141–150.

195. Sorscher SM, Dilsaver SC: Antidepressant-induced sexual dysfunction in men: Due to cholinergic blockade? *J Clin* Psychopharmacol. 6:53-55, 1986.

196. Gross MD: Reversal by bethanechol of sexual dysfunction caused by anticholinergic antidepressants. *Am J Psychiatry.* 139:1193-1194, 1982.

197. Gurwitz D, Lunshof JE, Dedoussis G *et al.*: Pharmacogenomics education: International Society of Pharmacogenomics recommendations for medical, pharmaceutical, and health schools deans of education. *Pharmacogenomics J.* 5, 221–225 (2005).

198. Dolgin, Ellie. Pharmacogenetic tests yield bonus benefit: better drug adherence. *Nature Medicine.* November, 2013 19 :11, 1354-5.

199. *The Case for Personalized Medicine* 4th edition 2014 (pmc@personalizedmedicinecoalition.org).

200. Zhang G, Zhang Y, Ling Y, Jia J. Web Resources for Pharmacogenomics. *Genomics Proteomics Bioinformatics* 13 (2015) 51–54.

201. Whirl-Carrillo M, McDonagh EM, Hebert JM, Gong L, Sangkuhl K, Thorn CF, et al. Pharmacogenomics knowledge for personalized medicine. *Clin Pharmacol Ther* 2012;92:414–7.

202. Law V, Knox C, Djoumbou Y, Jewison T, Guo AC, Liu Y, et al. DrugBank 4.0: shedding new light on drug metabolism. *Nucleic Acids Res* 2014;42:D1091–7.

203. Gamazon ER, Huang RS, Cox NJ. SCAN: a systems biology approach to pharmacogenomic discovery. *Methods Mol Biol* 2013;1015:213–24.

204. Gamazon ER, Duan S, Zhang W, Huang RS, Kistner EO, Dolan ME, et al. PACdb: a database for cell-based pharmacogenomics. *Pharmacogenet Genomics* 2010;20:269–73.

205. Garay MLG. The road from next-generation sequencing to personalized medicine. *Personalized Medicine* (2014) 11 (5), 523-544.

ABOUT THE AUTHORS

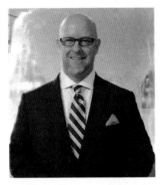

Dr. David Durham is a practicing neuropsychiatrist and a distinguished pharmacogenetics researcher. He completed his post-graduate medical training in psychiatric medicine at the University of Virginia and in neurocognitive electrophysiology at Duke University. He has a Master of Science in Public Health from the University of Kansas Medical Center and completed a research fellowship in ecological genetics at Benedictine College. He is an Assistant Clinical Professor of Psychiatry and Genomics, the current Chair of the Board of Governors of the American College of Neurocognitive Medicine and a clinical consultant to the United States Health and Human Services' IHS division. Dr. Durham is a recipient of the American College of Neurocognitive Medicine's Pioneer Investigator Award. He is a member of the scientific advisory board of Genelex Corporation, as well as the boards of directors of The Mosaic Group, Pangea Scientific LC and the United States Brain Injury Alliance (New Mexico). Dr. Durham has served as an editorial board member, review editor, and peer reviewer for a number of scientific journals and is a member of the American Neuropsychiatric Association, The International Neuropsychiatric Association, the International Society for Pharmacoeconomics and Outcomes Research, and the Clinical Pharmacogenetics Implementation Consortium. He is the former host of 'First Health with Dr. Dave' on Fox News.

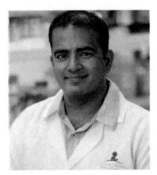

Dr. Ranjit Thirumaran is a distinguished researcher in pharmacogenetics, drug metabolism and genetic epidemiology. He earned his Master of Pharmacy at the Birla Institute of Technology - one of India's most prestigious institutions - and completed his Ph.D. in Molecular Genetic Epidemiology at the Ruprecht-Karls-Universität Heidelberg and German Cancer Research Center - Germany's largest biomedical research facility. He completed his post-doctoral fellowship in pharmacogenetics and drug metabolism and, thereafter, worked as a staff scientist at the prestigious St. Jude Children's Research Hospital in Memphis, Tennessee. He has published numerous scientific papers in a number of international research journals. Currently, Dr. Thirumaran is the Director of Clinical Pharmacogenetics at YouScript - an organization that has been a leader in precision medication management and clinical decision support analytics software that evaluates potential drug-drug and gene-drug interactions. Dr. Thirumaran has served as an editorial board member, review editor, and peer reviewer for a number of scientific journals and is a current/past member of the Association for Molecular Pathology, the American Pharmacists Association, the Clinical Pharmacogenetics Implementation Consortium, the American Society of Human Genetics, the International Society for the Study of Xenobiotics, and the Pharmacogenomics of Anticancer Agents Research Association.

Made in the USA
Lexington, KY
23 March 2017